Mechanisms of Environmental Carcinogenesis

Volume I

Role of Genetic and Epigenetic Changes

Editor

J. Carl Barrett

Head, Environmental Carcinogenesis Group
Laboratory of Pulmonary Pathobiology
National Institute of
Environmental Health Sciences
Research Triangle Park, North Carolina

CRC Press, Inc.
Boca Raton, Florida

Library of Congress Cataloging-in-Publication Data

Mechanisms of environmental carcinogenesis.

Contents: v. 1. Role of genetic and epigenetic
changes--v. 2. Multistep models of carcinogenesis.
Includes bibliographies and index.
1. Carcinogenesis. I. Barrett, J. Carl (James Carl)
[DNLM: 1. Carcinogens, Environmental--adverse effects.
2. Cell Transformation, Neoplastic--chemically induced.
3. Neoplasms, Experimental--chemically induced.
4. Neoplasms, Experimental--familial & genetic.
5. Oncogenes. QZ 202 M48547]
RC268.5.M436   1987   616.99′4071   86-34338
ISBN 0-8493-4670-3 (set)
ISBN 0-8493-4671-1 (v. 1)
ISBN 0-8493-4672-X (v. 2)

Direct all inquiries to CRC Press, Inc., 2000 Corporate Blvd., N.W., Boca Raton, Florida, 33431.

© 1987 by CRC Press, Inc.

International Standard Book Number 0-8493-4670-3 (Set)
International Standard Book Number 0-8493-4671-1 (Volume I)
International Standard Book Number 0-8493-4672-X (Volume II)
Library of Congress Card Number 86-34338
Printed in the United States

PREFACE

The process of neoplastic development is now recognized as a multistep process. Specific environmental chemicals can affect this process at unique stages suggesting the involvement of different mechanisms. Recent advances have been made in the understanding of the multistep process of carcinogenesis from experimental studies with animals and cells in culture. In addition, chemicals that affect specific stages of carcinogens have been identified from epidemiological studies of human cancer. The multistep process of carcinogenesis may involve multiple mechanism, epigenetic as well as genetic. The knowledge of the mechanisms of chemically induced genetic and nongenetic processes is to the point that the role of specific mechanisms in carcinogenesis can be discussed. This is exemplified by the study of viral and cellular oncogenes. These volumes present an overview of genetic and epigenetic processes in carcinogenesis. The multistep process of carcinogenesis is described and discussed in chapters on chemical carcinogenesis in animals, epidemiology of human cancers, cell transformation, and viral carcinogenesis. Further discussion of cellular and molecular mechanisms of carcinogenesis is presented in chapters dealing with tumor initiation, tumor promotion, and viral and cellular oncogenes. Examples of specific effects of chemicals and their mechanism of action in the multistep process of carcinogenesis are given and discussed. It is the objective of these volumes to outline possible cellular and molecular mechanisms of carcinogenesis in the context of a multistep process of neoplastic development and to relate these mechanisms to the effects of environmental substances.

THE EDITOR

J. Carl Barrett, Ph.D., is the head of the Environmental Carcinogenesis Group at the National Institute of Environmental Health Sciences, Research Triangle Park, North Carolina.

Dr. Barrett received his Ph.D. degree in Biophysical Chemistry at the Johns Hopkins University in 1974 and then spent 3 years as a postdoctoral fellow in the laboratory of Prof. Paul Ts'o at Johns Hopkins University. During that period he initiated his studies on the role of mutagenesis in carcinogenesis and the multistep process of neoplastic transformation of cells in culture. He has continued in this area and has made significant contributions to the understanding of the mechanisms of environmental carcinogenesis, such as asbestos, diethylstilbestrol, and arsenic, and to the cellular and molecular basis for the different stages on carcinogenesis. His current research efforts are focused on the study of oncogenes and tumor suppressor genes in neoplastic development.

CONTRIBUTORS

Volume I

J. Carl Barrett, Ph.D.
Chief
Environmental Carcinogenesis Section
National Institute of Environmental
  Health Sciences
Research Triangle Park, North
  Carolina

Timothy H. Carter, Ph.D.
Associate Professor
Department of Biological Sciences
St. John's University
Jamaica, New York

Nancy H. Colburn, Ph.D.
Chief, Cell Biology Section
Laboratory of Viral Carcinogenesis
National Cancer Institute
Frederick, Maryland

Peter A. Jones, Ph.D.
Director for Basic Science
Cancer Center
School of Medicine
University of Southern California
Los Angeles, California

Avery A. Sandberg, M.D.
Chief
Department of Genetics and
  Endocrinology
Roswell Park Memorial Institute
Buffalo, New York

Bernard E. Weissman, Ph.D.
Assistant Professor
Hematology/Oncology Division
Childrens Hospital of Los Angeles
Los Angeles, California

Gary M. Williams, M.D.
Associate Director, Naylor Dana
  Institute
Chief
Department of Pathology and
  Toxicology
American Health Foundation
Valhalla, New York

CONTRIBUTORS

Volume II

J. Carl Barrett, Ph.D.
Chief
Environmental Carcinogenesis Section
National Institute of Environmental
  Health Sciences
Research Triangle Park, North
  Carolina

Nicholas E. Day
Unit of Biostatistics
International Agency for Research on
  Cancer
Lyon, Cedex, France

Lennart C. Eriksson, M.D., Ph.D.
Associate Professor
Department of Pathology
Karolinska Institute
Stockholm, Sweden

Emmanuel Farber, M.D. Ph.D.
Professor
Departments of Pathology and
  Biochemistry
University of Toronto
Toronto, Ontario, Canada

William F. Fletcher, B.S.
Graduate Student
Laboratory for Pulmonary
  Pathobiology
Environmental Carcinogenesis Group
National Institute of Environmental
  Health Sciences
Research Triangle Park, North
  Carolina

Henry Hennings, Ph.D.
Research Chemist
Laboratory of Cellular Carcinogenesis
National Institutes of Health
National Cancer Institute
Bethesda, Maryland

John M. Kaldor, Ph.D.
Biostatistician
Unit of Biostatistics and Field Studies
Division of Epidemiology and
  Biostatistics
International Agency for Research on
  Cancer
Lyon, Cedex, France

Joel B. Rotstein, Ph.D.
Research Associate
Department of Pathology and
  Biochemistry
University of Toronto
Toronto, Ontario, Canada

TABLE OF CONTENTS

Volume I

Volume II

Chapter 1

GENETIC AND EPIGENETIC MECHANISMS OF CARCINOGENESIS

J. Carl Barrett

TABLE OF CONTENTS

I. INTRODUCTION

Cancer is the result of one or more heritable alterations in the tumor cell.[1] This fact was demonstrated nearly 50 years ago by Furth and Kahn,[2] who showed that the progeny of multiple single-cell clones from a tumor could reproduce the original disease upon reinjection of the cells into a suitable host. One of the fundamental questions facing cancer researchers is whether the nature of this heritable cellular alteration is genetic or epigenetic. This is not a new question; however, the recent identification of genetic alterations in specific oncogenes has provided new support for a genetic basis of cancer.[3] On the other hand, much data exist which are incompatible with a mutational theory of carcinogenesis.[4] In this chapter, I would like to summarize the lines of evidence for and against epigenetic vs. genetic alterations in carcinogenesis. In Chapter 13, Volume II, I will discuss possible models of carcinogenesis which encompass both mechanisms.

II. DEFINITIONS

Before discussing epigenetic and genetic mechanisms of carcinogenesis, it is necessary to discuss and define these and related terms since they have been used differently in different contexts. The term "epigenetic" was coined by Waddington[6] in 1940 to denote the "science concerned with the causal analysis of development". Waddington combined "epigenesis", the word used by William Harvey in the 17th century, to describe the development of the embryo from undifferentiated vital primorda, with genetics, which at that time was a new science actively under study by Waddington. Waddington proposed that development arose by what he termed an epigenetic process, to distinguish it from the preformation hypothesis. The discovery of the organizing region of the embryo by Spemann led Waddington[9] to propose the concept that a primary organizer in the embryo induces the formation of tissues or organs which later act as secondary organizers to drive further the epigenetic process of development.[6,8] According to Waddington's epigenetic hypothesis, the organizers produce substances (called evocators) which stimulate the cells to develop in response to this environmental signal. Waddington, however, also recognized the role of genetic factors in development *(Organizers and Genes* is the title of his classic book[6]), and he used the word "epigenotype",[9] to describe the epigenetic constitution of a certain piece of tissue or cell. The epigenotype represents the interaction of, among, and between genes and the external environment and is what contrasts different organs, such as the eye or nose, in an organism having a given genome.[10,11] The epigenotype is altered in transplantation experiments and results in altered development.[9]

With the understanding of the molecular biology of gene expression, the term epigenetic has also been used to describe processes related to the expression of genetic material by transcriptional and translational control mechanisms.[10] It is important in this context to distinguish genetic vs. epigenetic changes. Thus, the following definitions are used.

Epigenetic change — Any change in a phenotype which does not result from an alteration in DNA sequence. This change may be stable and heritable, and includes alterations in DNA methylation, transcriptional activation, translational control, and posttranslational modifications.

Genetic change — Any change in a phenotype which results from an alteration in primary DNA sequence. This change may be a single base pair change, a deletion, an insertion, a rearrangement or duplication of one or more base pairs, or loss or gain of an entire chromosome (Table 1) (genetic change = mutation).

Table 1
TYPES OF GENETIC CHANGES

1. Gene mutations (base substitution, frameshift mutations, deletion and insertion mutations)
2. Gene duplication or amplification (increased copies of a gene)
3. Chromosome aberrations (translocations, inversions, and deletions)
4. Aneuploidy (abnormal numbers of chromosomes)

Table 2
LINES OF EVIDENCE SUPPORTING SOMATIC MUTATION AS THE
BASIS FOR THE HERITABLE ALTERATION OF NEOPLASTIC CELLS
FOR THE HERITABLE ALTERATION OF NEOPLASTIC CELLS

1. Cancer is a heritable, stable change.
2. Tumors are generally clonal in nature.
3. Dominantly inherited tumors provide direct evidence for a genetic component in the origin of cancer.
4. Individuals who inherit recessive mutations associated with chromosome fragility or decreased DNA repair have increased cancer risks.
5. DNA is a critical target in carcinogenesis.
6. Carcinogens are mutagens.
7. Nonrandom chromosomal changes are associated with most cancers.
8. The transformed phenotype can be transferred from a tumor cell to a nontumor cell by DNA transfection.
9. Proto-oncogenes are activated by mutational mechanisms in tumor cells.

Confusion can arise from the use of the term epigenetic in the developmental context of Waddington and the molecular context of DNA structure. For example, the rearrangement of immunoglobulin genes during lymphocyte development is clearly a genetic change;[11] however, in the classical sense, this is an epigenetic change since it is related to the developmental process. The term "apogenetic",[12] which means associated with and deriving from genes, has been proposed to avoid this confusion. However, the word epigenetic is widely used to describe nongenetic changes in phenotype, and we will use this word as defined above in the following discussions.

III. EVIDENCE FOR GENETIC MECHANISMS IN CARCINOGENESIS

The origin of the somatic mutation theory of carcinogenesis is generally credited to Theodor Boveri, who in 1914 published his book entitled *Zur Frage der Entstehung Maligner Tumoren (On the Problem of the Origin of Malignant Tumors)*. The English translation of this book[13] by his wife, Marcella Boveri, was published in 1929. Boveri's hypothesis on the origin of malignant tumors was extraordinarily comprehensive and included many predictions which subsequently have been proven true. For these reasons, Boveri is generally acknowledged as the father of the somatic mutation theory of carcinogenesis. There is now considerable evidence to support his somatic mutation theory of carcinogenesis as outlined in Table 2 and discussed below.

Clearly, cancer is a stable, heritable cellular alteration. The classical experiments of Furth and Kahn[2] demonstrating this were mentioned earlier. Although stable, heritable traits occur by mutational changes, heritability per se is not proof of a mutational basis for a phenotype, since nonmutational mechanisms can also explain heritable changes.[14-16] Certain properties of differentiated cells are expressed as stable, heritable traits and have a nonmutational basis. Also, the stability of the malignant state is not absolute, and reversion of neoplasia can occur, which will be discussed in more detail in the next section.

The clonal origin of most tumors is also cited as evidence for the somatic mutation theory of carcinogenesis,[17] since a multiclonal tumor is inconsistent with the premise that a rare, genetic event is responsible for formation of a tumor. However, rare events may also have an epigenetic basis. Furthermore, the clonal appearance of a tumor only indicates that clonal selection has occurred, and a multiclonal tumor may become monoclonal by the time of detection.

Certain tumor syndromes are inherited dominantly with a high degree of penetrance.[17-20] One well-studied example of such syndromes is retinoblastoma. Persons who carry the gene for this disease have a 95% probability of developing retinoblastoma, and there is a 50% probability that their offspring will be carriers and will be affected. The individuals who carry this gene will be affected bilaterally, while noncarriers will often be affected only unilaterally. Knudson and others[17-20] have explained these observations on the basis of a two-hit model in which the expression of this tumor requires two steps to convert a normal cell into a neoplastic cell. In hereditary cases, the first step is an inherited, germ-line mutation and the second step, possibly a second mutation, occurs in a somatic cell. In the nonhereditary cases, two events are necessary in the somatic cell. Since only the second step is necessary in the hereditary case, the incidence is much higher than in the nonhereditary cases (95 in 100 vs. 1 in 20,000) and retinoblastoma occurs in both eyes.[17-20] Age-specific incidence data have provided substantial evidence that this disease occurs by two mutation-like steps. Recent molecular studies of retinoblastoma are consistent with this model; two mutations are required for expression of the retinoblastoma gene, a recessive human cancer gene which has a suppressor or regulatory function.[20]

There are other examples of familial cancers, including adenomatosis of the colon and rectum, which are inherited dominantly. Individuals with these genetic defects are predisposed to a high incidence of cancer in early life, consistent with an inheritance of at least one mutation necessary for neoplastic development.[21,22] Thus, dominantly inherited syndromes predisposing to neoplastic development provide direct evidence for a genetic component in the origin of cancer.

There are several observations which emphasize the importance of DNA damage in carcinogenesis. A number of cancer-prone, hereditary disorders including xeroderma pigmentosum, ataxia telangiectasia, Fanconi's anemia, Bloom's syndrome, and Cockayne's syndrome show abnormal cellular responses to DNA-damaging agents or have elevated spontaneous levels of chromosome rearrangements.[23,24] Furthermore, several lines of evidence indicate that DNA is a critical target for chemical carcinogens. The ultimate forms of most carcinogens are electrophiles which interact with DNA.[25] For certain chemicals, the extent of interaction with DNA correlates with carcinogenic potential, whereas the extent of carcinogen interaction with RNA or protein does not correlate with carcinogenicity;[26,27] however, it is difficult to identify specific DNA adducts which correlate with organ-specific carcinogenesis.[28]

Direct evidence for DNA as the critical target is provided by cell transformation experiments. Specific perturbations of DNA (for example, treatment of cells with 5-bromodeoxyuridine plus near-UV light, tritiated thymidine, or DNase encapsulated in liposomes) result in neoplastic transformation of Syrian hamster embryo cells in culture.[29-32] These results demonstrate that DNA is a susceptible target in carcinogenesis, since a specific perturbation directed at DNA is sufficient to induce neoplastic transformation. However, demonstration of DNA as a critical target does not rule out other potential non-DNA targets. Furthermore, these specific DNA perturbations may result in epigenetic changes by unknown mechanisms as well as genetic changes.

Significant experimental support for the somatic mutation theory of carcinogenesis was provided by the experiments of Ames and co-workers,[33,34] which suggested that

~90% of all carcinogens are mutagens. Despite this high apparent correlation between the mutagenicity and carcinogenicity of chemicals, several exceptions to this correlation exist.[35] Furthermore, this correlation decreases when one examines the mutagenicity of known human carcinogens.[35-37] Also, a recent review of mutagenicity in the Salmonella assay of chemicals tested for carcinogenicity in the bioassay program of the National Toxicology Program indicated that only 53% of the 130 carcinogens were mutagens, compared to 29% of 80 noncarcinogens.[38] Thus, a general correlation exists between mutagenicity and carcinogenicity, but the degree of correlation is considerably less than 100%; exceptions to this correlation exist and may indicate alternative mechanisms of carcinogenicity. This will be discussed in more detail in Chapter 8.

The most compelling evidence for a role of genetic changes in carcinogenicity comes from cytogenetic studies of tumors and molecular studies of oncogenes in neoplastic cells. Boveri's original somatic mutation theory was based on cytogenetic evidence.[13] Having observed that chromosomal aneuploidy resulted in developmental abnormalities, Boveri suggested a similar basis for the heritable alteration in malignant cells. He realized that tumors resulted from a cellular defect ("the problem of tumors is a cell problem"),[13] which he proposed prevents the normal control of cell proliferation, regulated by environmental (epigenetic) influences. Since control of developmental processes is very sensitive to chromosomal aberrations, Boveri proposed that "malignant tumors might be the result of a certain abnormal condition of the chromosomes." He believed that certain elements of the cell (chromosomes) could be disturbed without affecting cell viability. His theory emphasized chromosomal changes in malignant transformation and made no mention of point mutations. In 1928 Bauer expanded Boveri's theory to include mutations of genes.

With modern techniques of cytogenetics and molecular biology, the roles of chromosome changes in carcinogenesis have been well-documented. This area is covered extensively by Sandberg[40] in Chapter 6, in which he states hubristically that "a chromosome change is always at the root of cancer development." The number of cases which are the exceptions to this conclusion is decreasing with time.[40] The ubiquitous finding of nonrandom chromosome changes in tumors provides strong support for a genetic change in carcinogenesis. Also, when one examines the mutagenic activity of certain chemicals, a good correlation is observed with carcinogenicity and chromosome mutations.[41,42]

The identification of cellular oncogenes, their association with chromosomal rearrangements in tumors, and the demonstration of mutational mechanisms of activation of proto-oncogenes in certain tumors provide direct evidence for a genetic basis of carcinogenesis. Although the complete significance of oncogenes in the carcinogenesis process is still debated,[3,4,43-50] there is considerable evidence to support the conclusion that oncogenes are involved in certain steps of the neoplastic process. The finding that neoplastic potential can be transferred by transfection of DNA from tumor cells into nontumor cells demonstrates a genetic basis of these tumors.[45]

Studies on the molecular alterations of tumor or viral oncogenes vs. cellular proto-oncogenes provide insight into the type of mutational events involved in carcinogenesis. The proto-oncogenes of the *ras* family can be activated and can acquire transforming ability by a single point mutation (either a transition or a transversion) in the 12th or 61st codon.[3,44,45,51-54] The association of chromosome translocations with oncogene rearrangements is significant evidence for the importance of this type of genetic change in carcinogenesis. These rearrangements activate cellular oncogenes by either transcriptional or translational mechanisms.[3,40,49,50] Amplification of oncogenes occurs in a number of tumors, suggesting a role for this type of genetic change in the development or progression of malignancies.[49,55-59] Nonrandom numerical chromosomal changes

Table 3

LINES OF EVIDENCE SUPPORTING EPIGENETIC MECHANISMS AS THE BASIS FOR THE HERITABLE CHANGE IN NEOPLASTIC CELLS

1. Cancer is associated with altered differentiation and heritable changes occur during differentiation and development.
2. The cancerous state of tumor cells is sometimes reversible.
3. Some tumor cells have a diploid karyotype.
4. Carcinogenesis is induced by nonmutagenic treatments (such as plastic films and hormones).
5. Not all mutagens are carcinogens.
6. Carcinogenesis is associated with changes in DNA methylation.
7. Cell transformation can occur at very high frequencies.

are observed in many tumors. Trisomies of chromosomes with different oncogenes, particular *myc*, are observed in human and animal tumors.[40,60] Deletions of specific chromosomes are also observed.[40,60-63]

In summary, evidence for genetic changes on carcinogenesis comes from diverse studies of different aspects of carcinogenesis and mutagenesis. This evidence is quite compelling, and in some cases specific genetic changes at the molecular level have been pinpointed. However, evidence also exists for an epigenetic basis of carcinogenesis, and this will be reviewed in the next section.

IV. EVIDENCE FOR EPIGENETIC MECHANISMS IN CARCINOGENESIS

Several authors have noted numerous observations of cancer cells which are not easily explained on a genetic basis. Based on these observations, epigenetic mechanisms for carcinogenesis have been suggested.[1,4,14-16,25,31,43,64-67] Some of the lines of evidence supporting epigenetic mechanisms in carcinogenesis are listed in Table 3 and will be discussed below.

The most often cited argument for an epigenetic model of carcinogenesis is that the cancer problem is fundamentally an alteration in cellular differentiation, and the heritable cellular change responsible for the tumorigenic state is analogous to that which is involved in cell specialization during the normal course of development and differentiation.[64-68] The evidence for this hypothesis is based on (1) the heritability of cellular changes during differentiation and development, (2) the differentiated nature of many neoplasms, (3) the involvement of developmental genes in carcinogenesis, and (4) the reversibility of the neoplastic state.

It is quite clear that stable, heritable changes occur during development and differentiation[9,69,70] and, thus, the hypothesis that the cellular defect in carcinogenesis is an epigenetic alteration in normal growth control mechanisms is certainly valid. The differences between normal cells and tumors are not always great. Many of the fundamental characteristics of the cancer cell, including rapid cell division, migration, and invasion[68] are properties of some normal cells, and certainly occur during normal embryogenesis and development. Pierce and Cox[15] have referred to neoplasms as "caricatures of tissue renewal". Thus, the abnormality of cancer cells, i.e., unregulated cell growth, has long been postulated to result from a loss in the normal control processes of cell differentiation.

As more becomes known about the molecular defects in cancer cells, epigenetic mechanisms of altered gene expression in carcinogenesis may be elucidated. This possibility is increased by recent demonstrations of control of oncogene expression during normal cell development, differentiation, and proliferation.[73-83] Further studies in this

Table 4
EXAMPLES OF REVERSION OF NEOPLASTIC STATES

1. The neoplastic state of crown gall teratomas of tobacco plants can be reversibly suppressed.
2. Malignant mouse teratocarcinoma cells transplanted into blastocysts form normal, genetically mosaic mice.
3. Nuclear transplantation from renal tumors of the frog into ova develop normal tadpoles with no evidence of neoplasia.
4. Epidermoid carcinomas of the newt regress in the absence of the chemical inducer.
5. Spontaneous regression and differentiation of neuroblastomas of humans are observed occasionally.
6. Differentiation of squamous cell carcinoma cells is observed following transplantation.
7. Regression of chemically induced premalignant lesions (papillomas and dysplasias) frequently occurs.
8. Certain chemicals can induce terminal differentiation and/or reverse the neoplastic phenotype of malignant cells.
9. Cell-cell interactions and growth environment influence neoplastic and malignant potential of tumor cells.
10. Tumorigenicity can be suppressed in cell-cell hybrids and cybrids.
11. The reversion of the tumorigenic phenotype with a high frequency by carcinogens or agents such as 5-azacytidine affects patterns of DNA methylation.

area may provide concrete examples of epigenetic mechanisms in carcinogenesis, but these do not exist at present.

In some lower organisms, such as *Drosophilia melanogaster* and the ornamental swordtail fish (Xiphophorus), specific developmental or differentiation genes have been identified and shown to be involved in neoplasms of these species.[71,72] However, mutational mechanisms are involved in the heritable alterations in these genes in tumors. These model systems provide important lessons about the interaction of genetic and epigenetic mechanisms of carcinogenesis, which will be discussed in more detail in Chapter 13, Volume II.

One of the more important arguments in favor of an epigenetic basis for neoplasia is the ability to reverse the malignant state of some tumor cells. This phenomenon has been demonstrated in several experimental systems in response to a variety of treatments. Table 4 lists some of the experimental and spontaneous reversions of neoplastic states. Braun[66,84] has shown that the neoplastic state in cells of the crown gall teratomas of tobacco plants is completely but reversibly suppressed in plants grown from cloned cells. Whether the normal or tumor phenotype is expressed in the cells depends on activation or repression of certain biochemical signals.[84] Similarly, Mintz and co-workers[85,88] demonstrated elegantly that malignant murine teratocarcinoma cells can participate in normal development if injected into mouse blastocysts. Other examples of reversion or differentiation of malignant cells have been reported, including (1) the regression of epidermoid carcinoma in the newt produced by chemicals when the chemical stimulus is removed;[89] (2) spontaneous regression of neuroblastomas in humans; (3) differentiation of neuroblastoma of the tumor cells into morphologically normal adult neurons in vitro;[90,91] and (4) the loss of tumorigenicity and proliferative capacity of squamous cell carcinoma cells following differentiation.[15,92] In addition, premalignant lesions (papillomas and dysplasias) observed in several experimental models often regress with time and fail to progress to malignant lesions.[93-98]

Treatment of certain malignant cells with different chemical substances (e.g., retinoids, solvents, membrane active agents, base analogs, and interferon) will reverse the neoplastic phenotype of the cells, often by inducing cellular differentiation.[99-115] In addition, cell-cell interactions and the environment in which cells are grown can influence the properties of tumor cells. For example, the tumorigenicity of cells from preneoplastic mammary nodules is greatly enhanced by enzymatic dissociation and is reduced by the presence of normal mammary cells.[116] The stability of the metastatic phenotype of murine melanoma cells is greatly affected by cellular interactions,[117] and the malignant phenotype of a human carcinoma cell line is expressed or lost depending on the physiological environment in which the cells are maintained.[118]

Suppression of malignancy has also been observed in hybrids formed by fusion of some, but not all, malignant cells with normal cells.[119-130] Suppression of tumorigenicity may be controlled by genetic factors since the presence of specific chromosomes is required in some hybrids for suppression,[131-135] or by epigenetic factors since the cytoplasm alone can suppress tumorigenicity of certain normal cells.[136-140]

As can be seen from the preceding discussion, the suppression or reversion of the neoplastic and malignant state can be affected by a variety of epigenetic influences. However, as discussed by Harris[119] some years ago, this "does not, however, constitute evidence for the view that malignancy is determined by epigenetic mechanisms." He discussed the crown gall tumor example and noted that this tumor is caused by a genetic change, i.e., the insertion of a plasmid carried by the tumorigenic bacterium, *Agrobacterium tumefacians,* and evidence exists that this plasmid contains genetic information responsible for the transformation of the plant cells.[119] Harris offers as an alternative explanation for these observations of tumor suppression or reversion that "the malignant phenotype may be suppressed, or held in abeyance, by the process of differentiation." Thus, a heritable, genetic alteration may occur in, and be responsible for, the neoplastic change(s) in a tumor, and yet this cell may be suppressed by an epigenetic mechanism resulting from differentiation or some other mechanism of growth arrest.

Recent experimental results illustrate that such suppressive mechanisms can occur in cells with defined genetic alterations responsible for the neoplastic state. For example, upon treatment of HL-60 leukemia and other cells with inducers of differentiation, growth arrest and decreased expression of the c-*myc* gene occur even though this oncogene is amplified or rearranged;[141-146] the translocated c-*myc* oncogene is also repressed in certain cell hybrids;[147-151] and the tumorigenicity of cells transformed by the mutated EJ-*ras* oncogene is suppressed in cell-cell hybrids even though the *ras* gene is still expressed.[152] Thus, some authors have proposed that antioncogenes exist which suppress tumorigenicity by unknown mechanisms.[152]

Other lines of evidence for epigenetic mechanisms of carcinogenesis include the observations that some tumors have a diploid karyotype, not all carcinogens are mutagenic, and not all mutagens are carcinogens. The ubiquitous finding of karyotypic changes in tumors was discussed earlier in this chapter and Chapter 6. The finding of diploid tumors is exceptional and may be due to the presence of normal cells within the tumor; furthermore, submicroscopic genetic alterations may be present in apparently diploid tumors.[40] Multiple explanations can be offered for apparent exceptions to the correlation of mutagenicity and carcinogenicity. Difficulties arise when one compares carcinogenicity in vivo with mutagenicity in some other target cell, generally in vitro. Differences in metabolic activation, DNA adduct formation and repair, and pharmacokinetics can give rise to apparent differences. Also, some previously considered nonmutagenic carcinogenic insults, such as asbestos fibers and hormones, may have mutagenic activities (see Chapters 8, this volume, and Chapter 12, Volume II). The relationship between mutagenicity and carcinogenicity is a complicated area which will be discussed separately in Chapter 8.

One epigenetic mechanism in carcinogenesis which is receiving recent support is altered gene expression arising from changes in DNA methylation. As is discussed in more detail in Chapter 2, evidence for a role of this mechanism is now available in at least some steps in carcinogenesis.

It is often assumed[64] that if neoplastic transformation is the result of a rare genetic change, then the frequency of this change should be very low, for example, 1 in 10^5 or

1 in 10⁶. However, the frequency of cell transformation in vitro has been reported to be very high, in some cases approaching unity.[155-160] These results have been interpreted as evidence for an epigenetic rather than a genetic mechanism of carcinogenesis.[64] However, caution must be exercised in interpreting these results.[153-159] In some cases, the frequency noted is not the actual frequency of transformed cells in the population, but rather the frequency of induction or activation of the cells which leads to the transformation by a two-step mechanism, i.e., carcinogen treatment of small numbers (one to five) of certain cells activates the cells by an unknown mechanism and increases the probability that the progeny of these activated cells will transform. This second, transforming step occurs with much lower frequency consistent with a possible mutational mechanism.[153,157,159,161] In systems using primary cell cultures, a relatively high frequency of transformation ($\sim 1\%$) is directly induced; however, this alteration may be explained by a mutational event if the number of target genes is large, if a mutational hotspot exists, or if the mutation is a chromosomal event.[153,159,160] Thus, the measurement of frequency alone does not distinguish genetic from epigenetic mechanisms.

V. CONCLUSION

I have reviewed a wide variety of observations supporting genetic or epigenetic mechanisms for carcinogenesis. Strong support for both hypotheses exist, and further discussion of these mechanisms is presented throughout this book. It has not been shown in any tumor model that only a genetic or epigenetic mechanism is involved. The reasons for this are clear; carcinogenesis is a multistep, multicausal, multigenic process (see Chapter 13, Volume II). Both genetic and epigenetic forces are involved in the progression of this disease. With the current advances in molecular biology, the interplay of genetic and epigenetic factors in carcinogenesis is beginning to be understood. It is the intended purpose of this book, therefore, not to resolve whether genetic *or* epigenetic changes are involved in carcinogenesis, but rather to illustrate interesting biological aspects of the carcinogenic process which will be useful in future studies of the mechanisms and causes of this disease and possible means to interfere with its development and progression.

REFERENCES

1. Barrett, J. C., Crawford, B. D., and Ts'o, P. O. P., The role of somatic mutation in a multistage model of carcinogenesis, in *Mammalian Cell Transformation by Chemical Carcinogens,* Dunkel, V. C. and Mishra, R. A., Eds., Pathox Publishing, New York, 1980, 467.
2. Furth, J. and Kahn, M. C., The transmission of leukemia of mice with a single cell, *Am. J. Cancer,* 31, 276, 1937.
3. Varmus, H. E., The molecular genetics of cellular oncogenes, *Annu. Rev. Genet.,* 18, 553, 1984.
4. Rubin, H., Cancer as a dynamic developmental disorder, *Cancer Res.,* 45, 2935, 1985.
5. Barrett, J. C., A multistep model for neoplastic development: role of genetic and epigenetic changes, in *Mechanisms of Environmental Carcinogenesis,* Vol. 2, Barrett, J. C., Ed., CRC Press, Boca Raton, Fla., 1987, chap. 13.
6. Waddington, C. H., *Organizers and Genes,* Cambridge University Press, London, 1940.
7. Waddington, C. H., *The Epigenetics of Birds,* Cambridge University Press, London, 1952.
8. Ede, D. A., *An Introduction to Developmental Biology,* John Wiley & Sons, New York, 1978.
9. Waddington, C. H., *An Introduction to Modern Genetics,* Allen and Urwin, London, 1939.
10. Rieger, R., Michaelis, A., and Green, M. M., *A Glossary of Genetics and Cytogenetics — Classical and Molecular,* Springer-Verlag, New York, 1976.

11. Baltimore, D., Somatic mutation gains its place among the generators of diversity, *Cell,* 127, 295, 1981.
12. Sibatani, A., Epigenetic and apogenetic, *Riv. Biol.,* 76, 657, 1983.
13. Boveri, T. H., *The Origin of Malignant Tumors,* Williams & Wilkins, Baltimore, 1929.
14. Mintz, B., Genetic mosaicism and *in vitro* analysis of neoplasia and differentiation, in *Cell Differentiation and Neoplasia,* Saunders, G. F., Ed., Raven Press, New York, 1978, 27.
15. Pierce, G. B. and Cox, W. F., Neoplasms as caricatures of tissue renewal, in *Cell Differentiation and Neoplasia,* Saunders, G. F., Ed., Raven Press, New York, 1978, 57.
16. Weinstein, I. B., Yamaguchi, N., Gebert, R., and Kaighn, M. E., Use of epithelial cell cultures for studies on the mechanism of transformation by chemical carcinogens, *In Vitro,* 11, 130, 1975.
17. Knudson, A. G., Mutation and human cancer, *Adv. Cancer Res.,* 17, 317, 1973.
18. Knudson, A. G., Hethcote, H. W., and Brown, B. W., Mutation and childhood cancer: a probabilistic model for the incidence of retinoblastoma, *Proc. Natl. Acad. Sci. U.S.A.,* 72, 5116, 1975.
19. Hethcote, H. W. and Knudson, A. G., Model for the incidence of embryonal cancers: application to retinoblastoma, *Proc. Natl. Acad. Sci. U.S.A.,* 75, 2453, 1978.
20. Murphee, A. L. and Benedict, W. F., Retinoblastoma: clues to human oncogenesis, *Science,* 223, 1028, 1984.
21. Mulvihill, J. J., Genetic repertory of human neoplasia, in *Genetics of Human Cancer,* Mulvihill, J. J., Miller, R. W., and Fraumeni, J. F., Eds., Raven Press, New York, 1977, 137.
22. Lipkin, M. and Deschner, E. E., Gastrointestinal neoplasia: an investigative approach, in *Genetics of Human Cancer,* Mulvihill, J. J., Miller, R. W., and Fraumeni, J. F., Eds., Raven Press, New York, 1977, 369.
23. German, J., Genes which increase chromosomal instability in somatic cells and predispose to cancer, in *Progress in Medical Genetics,* Vol. 8, Steinberg, A. G. and Bearn, A. G., Eds., Grune & Stratton, New York, 1972, 61.
24. Arlett, C. F. and Lehmann, A. R., Human disorders showing increased sensitivity to induction of genetic damage, *Annu. Rev. Genet.,* 12, 95, 1978.
25. Miller, E. C. and Miller, J. A., The mutagenicity of chemical carcinogens: correlations, problems and interpretations, in *Chemical Mutagenesis Principles & Methods for their Detection,* Vol. 1, Hollaender, A., Ed., Plenum Press, New York, 1971, 83.
26. Brookes, P., Quantitative aspects of the reaction of some carcinogens with nucleic acids and the possible significance of such reactions in the process of carcinogenesis, *Cancer Res.,* 26, 1994, 1966.
27. Brookes, P. and Lawley, P. D., Evidence for the binding of polynuclear aromatic hydrocarbons to the nucleic acids of mouse skin: relation between carcinogenic power of hydrocarbons and their binding to deoxyribonucleic acid, *Nature (London),* 202, 781, 1964.
28. Rajewsky, M. F., Possible determinants for the differential susceptibility of mammalian cells and tissues to chemical carcinogenesis, in *Quantitative Aspects of Risk Assessment in Chemical Carcinogenesis,* Clemmensen, J., Ed., Springer-Verlag, New York, 1980, 229.
29. Barrett, J. C., Tsutsui, T., and Ts'o, P. O. P., Neoplastic transformation induced by a direct perturbation of DNA, *Nature (London),* 274, 229, 1978.
30. Tsutsui, T., Barrett, J. C., and Ts'o, P. O. P., Chromosomal aberrations, DNA damage and morphological transformation of synchronized Syrian hamster embryo cells: effect of 5-bromodeoxyuridine and near ultraviolet radiation, *Cancer Res.,* 39, 2356, 1979.
31. Bruce, S. A., Gyi, K. K., Nakano, S., Ueo, H., Zajac-Kaye, M., and Ts'o, P. O. P., Genetic and developmental determinants in neoplastic transformation, in *Biochemical Basis of Chemical Carcinogenesis,* Griem, H., Jung, R., Kramer, K., Marquardt, H., and Oesch, F., Eds., Raven Press, New York, 1984, 159.
32. Zajac-Kaye, M. and Ts'o P. O. P., DNase I encapsulated in liposomes can induce neoplastic transformation of Syrian hamster embryo cells in culture, *Cell,* 39, 427, 1984.
33. McCann, J. and Ames, B. N., Detection of carcinogens as mutagens in the Salmonella/microsome test: assay of 300 chemicals. Discussion, *Proc. Natl. Acad. Sci. U.S.A.,* 72, 950, 1976.
34. McCann, J., Choi, E., Yamasaki, E., and Ames, B. N., Detection of carcinogens as mutagens in the Salmonella/microsome test: assay of 300 chemicals, *Proc. Natl. Acad. Sci. U.S.A.,* 72, 5135, 1975.
35. Barrett, J. C., Hesterberg, T. W., and Thomassen, D. G., Use of cell transformation systems for carcinogenicity testing and mechanistic studies of carcinogenesis, *Pharmacol. Rev.,* 36, 53S, 1984.
36. Garrett, N. E., Stack, H. F., Gross, M. R., and Waters, M. D., An analysis of the spectra of genetic activity produced by known or suspected human carcinogens, *Mutat. Res.,* 134, 89, 1984.
37. Williams, G. M., DNA reactive and epigenetic carcinogens, in *Mechanisms of Environmental Carcinogenesis,* Vol. 1, Barrett, J. C., Ed., CRC Press, Boca Raton, Fla., 1987, chap. 7.
38. Zeiger, E. and Tennant, R. W., Mutagenesis, clastogenesis, carcinogenesis: expectations, correlations and relations, in *Genetic Toxicology of Environmental Chemicals, Part B: Genetic Effects and Applied Mutagenesis,* Ramel, C., Lambert, B., and Magnusson, J., Eds., Alan R. Liss, New York, 1986, 75.

39. Barrett, J. C., Relationship between mutagenesis and carcinogenesis, in *Mechanisms of Environmental Carcinogenesis,* Vol. 1, Barrett, J. C., Ed., CRC Press, Boca Raton, Fla., 1987, chap. 8.
40. Sandberg, A. A., Role of chromosome changes in carcinogenesis, in *Mechanisms of Environmental Carcinogenesis,* Vol. 1, Barrett, J. C., Ed., CRC Press, Boca Raton, Fla., 1987, chap. 6.
41. Ishidate, M. and Odashima, S., Chromosome tests with 134 compounds on Chinese hamster cells *in vitro.* A screening for chemical carcinogens, *Mutat. Res.,* 48, 337, 1977.
42. Barrett, J. C., Thomassen, D. G., and Hesterberg, T. W., Role of gene and chromosomal mutations in cell transformation, *Ann. N.Y. Acad. Sci.,* 407, 291, 1983.
43. Rubin, H., Mutations and oncogenes — cause or effect?, *Nature (London),* 309, 518, 1984.
44. Bishop, J. M., Cellular oncogenes and retroviruses, *Annu. Rev. Biochem.,* 52, 301, 1983.
45. Weinberg, R. A., Oncogenes of spontaneous and chemically induced tumors, *Adv. Cancer Res.,* 36, 149, 1982.
46. Duesberg, P. H., Retroviral transforming genes in normal cells?, *Nature (London),* 304, 219, 1983.
47. Duesberg, P. H., Activated proto-oncogenes: sufficient or necessary for cancer?, *Science,* 228, 669, 1985.
48. Land, H., Parada, L. F., and Weinberg, R. A., Cellular oncogenes and multistep carcinogenesis, *Science,* 222, 771, 1983.
49. Klein, G. and Klein, E., Oncogene activation and tumor progression, *Carcinogenesis,* 5, 429, 1984.
50. Croce, C. M., Gene regulation in the expression of malignancy, *Cancer Surv.,* 3, 287, 1984.
51. Reddy, E. P., Reynolds, R. K., Santos, E., and Barbacid, M., Point mutation is responsible for the acquisition of transforming properties by the T24 human bladder carcinoma oncogene, *Nature (London),* 300, 149, 1982.
52. Tabin, C. J., Bradley, S. M., Bargmann, C. I., and Weinberg, R. A., Papageorge, A. G., Scolnick, E. M., Dhar, R., Lowy, D. R., and Chang, E. H., Mechanism of activation of a human oncogene, *Nature (London),* 300, 143, 1982.
53. Yuasa, Y., Srivastara, S. K., Dunn, G. Y., Rhim, J. S., Reddy, E. P., and Aaronson, S. A., Acquisition of transforming properties by alternative point mutations within c-bas/has human proto-oncogene, *Nature (London),* 303, 775, 1983.
54. Zarbl, H., Sukumar, S., Martin-Zanca, D., Santos, E., and Barbacid, M., Molecular assays for detection of *ras* oncogenes on human and animal tumors, in *Carcinogenesis: A Comprehensive Survey,* Vol. 9, Barrett, J. C. and Tennant, R. W., Eds., Raven Press, New York, 1985, 1.
55. Brodeur, G. M., Seeger, R. C., Schwab, M., Varmus, H. E., and Bishop, J. M., Amplification of N-myc in untreated human neuroblastomas correlates with advanced-disease stage, *Science,* 224, 1121, 1984.
56. Little, C. D., Nou, M. M., Carney, D. N., Gazdar, A. F., and Minna, J. D., Amplification and expression of the c-myc oncogene in human lung cancer cell lines, *Nature (London),* 306, 194, 1983.
57. Schwab, M., Alitalo, K., Klempnauer, K. H., Varmus, H. E., Bishop, J. M., Gilbert, F., Brodeur, G., Goldstein, M., and Trent, J., Amplified DNA with limited homology to myc cellular oncogene is shared by human neuroblastoma cell lines and a neuroblastoma tumor, *Nature (London),* 305, 245, 1983.
58. Nowell, P., Finan, J., Favera, R. D., Gallo, R. C., Ar-Rushdi, A., Romanezuk, H., Selden, J. R., Emanuel, B. S., Rovera, G., and Croce, C. M., Association of amplified oncogene c-myc with an abnormally banded chromosome and in a human leukemic cell line, *Nature (London),* 306, 494, 1983.
59. Favera, R. D., Wong-Staal, F., and Gallo, R. C., Oncogene amplification in promyelocytic leukemia cell line HL-60 and primary leukemic cells of the same patient, *Nature (London),* 299, 61, 1982.
60. Oshimura, M. and Barrett, J. C., Chemically induced aneuploidy in mammalian cells — mechanisms and significance in cancer, *Environ. Mutagenesis,* 8, 129, 1986.
61. Murphree, A. L. and Benedict, W. F., Retinoblastoma: clues to human oncogenesis, *Science,* 223, 1028, 1984.
62. Cavenee, W. K., Dryja, T. P., Phillips, R. A., Benedict, W. F., Godbout, R., Gallie, B. L., Murphree, A. L., Strong, L. C., and White, R. L., Expression of recessive alleles by chromosomal mechanisms in retinoblastoma, *Nature (London),* 305, 779, 1983.
63. Koufos, A., Hansen, M. F., Copeland, N. G., Jenkins, N. A., Hampkin, B. C., and Cavenee, W. K., Loss of heterozygosity in three embryonal tumors suggests a common pathogenetic mechanism, *Nature (London),* 316, 330, 1985.
64. Rubin, H., Is somatic mutation the major mechanism of malignant transformation?, *J. Natl. Cancer Inst.,* 64, 995, 1980.
65. Pitot, H. C., Neoplasia — a somatic mutation or a heritable change in cytoplasmic membrane?, *J. Natl. Cancer Inst.,* 53, 905, 1974.
66. Braun, A. C., An epigenetic model for the origin of cancer, *Q. Rev. Biol.,* 56, 33, 1981.
67. Frost, P. and Kerbel, R. S., On a possible epigenetic mechanism(s) of tumor cell heterogeneity, *Cancer Metastasis Rev.,* 2, 375, 1978.

68. Markert, C. L., Neoplasmia: a disease of cell differentiation, *Cancer Res.,* 28, 1908, 1968.
69. Jeffery, W. R., Specification of cell fate by cytoplasmic determinants in Ascidian embryos, *Cell,* 41, 11, 1985.
70. DiBerardino, M. A., Hoffner, N. J., and Laurence, E. D., Activation of dormant genes in specialized cells, *Science,* 224, 946, 1984.
71. Gateff, E., Malignant neoplasms of genetic origin in *Drosophilia melanogaster, Science,* 200, 1448, 1978.
72. Anders, F., Schartl, M., Barnekow, A., and Anders, A., *Xiphophorus* as an *in vivo* model for studies on normal and defective control of oncogenes, *Adv. Cancer Res.,* 42, 191, 1984.
73. Yaswen, P., Goyette, M., Shank, P. R., and Fausto, N., Expression of c-Ki-ras, c-Ha-ras, and c-myc in specific cell types during hepatocarcinogenesis, *Mol. Cell. Biol.,* 5, 780, 1985.
74. Leder, P., Batlery, J., Lenoir, G., Moulding, C., Murphy, W., Potter, H., Stewart, T., and Taub, R., Translocation among antibody genes in human cancer, *Science,* 222, 765, 1983.
75. Kruijer, W., Copper, J. A., Hunter, T., and Verma, I. M., Platelet-derived growth factor induced rapid but transient expression of the c-fos gene and protein, *Nature (London),* 312, 711, 1984.
76. Müller, R., Bravo, R., Burckhardt, J., and Curran, T., Induction of c-fos gene and protein by growth factors precedes activation of c-myc, *Nature (London),* 312, 716, 1984.
77. Pfeifer-Ohlsson, S., Goustin, A., Rydnert, J., Wahlstron, T., Bjersing, L., Stehelin, D., and Ohlsson, R., Spatial and temporal pattern of cellular myc oncogene expression in developing human placenta: implication for embryonic cell proliferation, *Cell,* 38, 585, 1984.
78. Jaye, M., McConathy, E., Drohan, W., Tong, B., Devel, T., and Maciag, T., Modulation of the sis gene transcript during endothelial cell differentiation *in vitro, Science,* 228, 882, 1985.
79. Müller, R., Slamon, D. J., Adamson, E. D., Tremblay, J. M., Müller, D., Cline, M. J., and Verma, I. M., Transcription of c-onc genes c-ras^{Ki} and c-fms during mouse development, *Mol. Cell. Biol.,* 3, 1062, 1983.
80. Goustin, A. S., Betsholtz, C., Pfeifer-Ohlsson, S., Persson, H., Rydnert, J., Bywater, M., Holmgren, G., Heldin, C-H., Westermark, B., and Ohlson, R., Coexpression of the sis and myc protooncogene in developing human placenta suggests autocrine control of trophoblast growth, *Cell,* 41, 301, 1985.
81. Fausto, N. and Shank, P. R., Oncogene expression in liver regeneration and hepatocarcinogenesis, *Hepatology,* 3, 1016, 1983.
82. Slamon, D. J. and Cline, M. J., Expression of cellular oncogenes during embryonic and fetal development of the mouse, *Proc. Natl. Acad. Sci. U.S.A.,* 83, 7141, 1984.
83. Müller, R., Slamon, D. J., Tremblay, J. M., Cline, M. J., and Verma, I. M., Differential expression of cellular oncogenes during pre- and postnatal development of the mouse, *Nature (London),* 299, 640, 1982.
84. Braun, A. C. and Wood, H. N., Suppression of the neoplastic state with the acquisition of specialized function in cells, tissues, and organs of crown gall teratomas of tobacco, *Proc. Natl. Acad. Sci. U.S.A.,* 73, 496, 1976.
85. Mintz, B. and Illmensee, K., Normal genetically mosaic mice produced from malignant teratocarcinoma cells, *Proc. Natl. Acad. Sci. U.S.A.,* 72, 3585, 1975.
86. Illmensee, K. and Mintz, B., Totipotency and normal differentiation of single teratocarcinoma cells cloned by injection into blastocysts, *Proc. Natl. Acad. Sci. U.S.A.,* 73, 549, 1976.
87. Stewart, T. A. and Mintz, B., Successive generations of mice produced from an established culture line of euploid teratocarcinoma cells, *Proc. Natl. Acad. Sci. U.S.A.,* 78, 6314, 1981.
88. Mintz, B. and Fleischman, R. A., Teratocarcinomas and other neoplasms as developmental defects in gene expression, in *Advances in Cancer Research,* Vol. 34, Weinhouse, S. and Klein, G., Eds., Academic Press, New York, 1981, 211.
89. Seilern-Aspang, F. and Kratochwil, K., Induction and differentiation of an epithelial tumor in the newt (Triturus cristatus), *J. Embryol. Exp. Morphol.,* 10, 337, 1962.
90. Goldstein, M. N., Burdman, J. A., and Journey, L. J., Long-term tissue culture of neuroblastomas: morphological evidence for differentiation and maturation, *J. Natl. Cancer Inst.,* 32, 165, 1964.
91. Prasad, K. N. and Sinha, P. K., *Cell Differentiation and Neoplasia,* Saunders, G. F., Ed., Raven Press, New York, 1978, 111.
92. Pierce, G. B. and Wallace, C., Differentiation of malignant to benign cell, *Cancer Res.,* 32, 127, 1971.
93. Burns, F. J., Vanderlaan, M., Sivak, A., and Albert, R. E., Regression kinetics of mouse skin papillomas, *Cancer Res.,* 36, 1422, 1976.
94. Nettesheim, P., Klein-Szanto, A. J. P., Morchok, A. C., Steele, V. E., Terzaghi, M., and Topping, D. C., Studies of neoplastic development in respiratory tract epithelium, *Arch. Pathol. Lab. Med.,* 105, 1, 1981.

95. Griesemer, R. A., Nettesheim, P., and Marchok, A. C., Fate of early carcinogen-induced lesions in tracheal epithelium, *Cancer Res.*, 36, 2659, 1976.
96. Topping, D. C., Pal, B. C., Martin, D. H., Nelson, F. R., and Nettesheim, P., Pathologic changes induced in respiratory tract mucosa by polycyclic hydrocarbons of differing carcinogen activity, *Am. J. Pathol.*, 93, 311, 1978.
97. Nettesheim, P., Griesemer, R. A., Martin, D. H., and Caton, J. E., Jr., Induction of preneoplastic and neoplastic lesions in grafted rat tracheas continuously exposed to benzo(a)pyrene, *Cancer Res.*, 37, 1271, 1977.
98. Topping, D. C., Griesemer, R. A., and Nettesheim, P., Development and fate of focal epithelial lesions in tracheal mucosa following exposure to 7,12-dimethylbenz(a)anthracene, *Cancer Res.*, 39, 4829, 1979.
99. Sporn, M. B. and Roberts, A. B., Role of retinoids in differentiation and carcinogenesis, *Cancer Res.*, 43, 3034, 1983.
100. Fraker, L. D., Halter, S. A., and Forbes, J. T., Growth inhibition by retinol of a human breast carcinoma cell line *in vitro* and in athymic mice, *Cancer Res.*, 44, 5757, 1984.
101. Gensler, H. L., Matrisian, L. M., and Bowden, G. T., Effect of retinoic acid on the late-stage promotion of transformation in JB6 mouse epidermal cells in culture, *Cancer Res.*, 45, 1922, 1985.
102. Ong, D. F. and Chytil, F., Vitamin A and cancer, in *Vitamins and Hormones*, Vol. 40, Academic Press, New York, 1983, 105.
103. Jetten, A. M., Jetten, M. E. R., and Sherman, M. I., Stimulation of differentiation of several murine embryonal carcinoma cell lines by retinoic acid, *Exp. Cell Res.*, 124, 381, 1979.
104. Merriman, R. L. and Bertram, J. S., Reversible inhibition by retinoids of 3-methylcholanthrene-induced neoplastic transformation in C3H/10T$_{1/2}$ clone 8 cells, *Cancer Res.*, 39, 1661, 1979.
105. Strickland, S. and Mahdari, V., The induction of differentiation in teratocarcinoma stem cells by retinoic acid, *Cell*, 15, 293, 1978.
106. Dion, L. D., Blalock, J. E., and Gifford, G. E., Retinoic acid and the restoration of anchorage dependent growth to transformed mammalian cells, *Exp. Cell Res.*, 117, 15, 1978.
107. Jetten, A. M. and Jetten, M. E. R., Possible role of retinoic acid binding protein in retinoid stimulation of embryonal carcinoma cell differentiation, *Nature (London)*, 278, 180, 1979.
108. Honma, V., Tokenaga, K., Kasukabe, T., and Hozumi, M., Induction of differentiation of cultured human promyelocytic leukemia cells by retinoids, *Biochem. Biophys. Res. Commun.*, 95, 507, 1980.
109. Bodner, A. J., Ting, R. C., and Gallo, R. C., Induction of differentiation of human promyelocytic leukemia cells (HL-60) by nucleosides and methotrexate, *J. Natl. Cancer Inst.*, 67, 1025, 1981.
110. Nomura, S. and Oishi, M., Indirect induction of erythroid differentiation in mouse friend cells: evidence for two intracellular reactions involved in the differentiation, *Proc. Natl. Acad. Sci. U.S.A.*, 80, 210, 1983.
111. Scher, W., Tsuei, D., Sassa, S., Price, P., Gabelman, N., and Friend, C., Inhibition of dimethylsulf-oxide-stimulated friend cells erythroid differentiation by hydrocortisone and other steroids, *Proc. Natl. Acad. Sci. U.S.A.*, 75, 3851, 1978.
112. Gosella, J. F. and Housman, D., Induction of erythroid differentiation *in vitro* by purines and purine analogues, *Cell*, 8, 263, 1976.
113. Nakayasu, M., Terada, M., Tamura, G., and Sugimura, T., Induction of differentiation of human and murine myeloid leukemia cells in culture by tunicamycin, *Proc. Natl. Acad. Sci. U.S.A.*, 77, 409, 1980.
114. Marquardt, H., The mechanisms of chemically induced malignant transformation: its inhibition by polynucleotides and its reversion by 5-bromodeoxyuridine, in *Biochemical Basis of Chemical Carcinogenesis*, Greim, H., Jung, R., Kramer, M., Marquardt, H., and Oesh, F., Eds., Raven Press, New York, 1984, 189.
115. Brouty-Boye, D., Wybier-Franqui, J., Calvo, C., Feunteun, J., and Gresser, I., Reversibility of the transformed and neoplastic phenotype: effects of long-term interferon treatment of C3H/10T$_{1/2}$ cells transformed by methylcholanthrene and SV40 virus, *Int. J. Cancer*, 34, 107, 1984.
116. Medina, D., Shepherd, F., and Gropp, T., Enhancement of the tumorigenicity of preneoplastic mammary nodule lines by enzymatic dissociation, *J. Natl. Cancer Inst.*, 60, 1121, 1978.
117. Poste, G., Doll, J., and Fidler, I. J., Interactions among clonal subpopulation affects stability of the metastatic phenotype in polyclonal populations of B16 melanoma cells, *Proc. Natl. Acad. Sci. U.S.A.*, 78, 6226, 1981.
118. Ossowski, L. and Reich, E., Changes in malignant phenotype of a human carcinoma conditioned by growth environment, *Cell*, 33, 323, 1983.
119. Harris, H., Some thoughts about genetics, differentiation and malignancy, *Somat. Cell Genet.*, 5, 923, 1979.
120. Barski, G. and Belehrader, J., Jr., Inheritance of malignancy in somatic cell hybrids, *Somat. Cell Genet.*, 5, 897, 1979.

121. Klinger, H. P., Suppression of tumorigenicity in somatic cell hybrids, *Cytogenet. Cell Genet.*, 27, 254, 1980.
122. Stanbridge, E. J., Suppression of malignancy in human cells, *Nature (London)*, 260, 17, 1976.
123. Stanbridge, E. J. and Wilkinson, J., Analysis of malignancy in human cells: malignant and transformed phenotypes are under separate genetic control, *Proc. Natl. Acad. Sci. U.S.A.*, 75, 1466, 1978.
124. Weissman, B. E. and Stanbridge, E. J., Complementation of the tumorigenic phenotype in human cell hybrids, *J. Natl. Cancer Inst.*, 70, 667, 1983.
125. Stanbridge, E. J., Der, C. J., Doersen, C. J., Nishimi, R. Y., Peehl, D. M., Weissman, B. E., and Wilkinson, J. E., Human cell hybrids: analysis of transformation and tumorigenicity, *Science*, 25, 252, 1982.
126. Sager, R. and Korac, P. E., Genetic analysis of tumorigenesis: chromosome reduction and marker segregation in progeny clones from Chinese hamster cell hybrids, *Somat. Cell Genet.*, 5, 491, 1979.
127. Marshall, C. J. and Sager, R., Genetic analysis of tumorigenesis: suppression of anchorage independence in hybrids between transformed hamster cell lines, *Somat. Cell Genet.*, 7, 713, 1981.
128. Croce, C. M., Barrick, J., Linnenbach, A., and Koprowski, H., Expression of malignancy in hybrids between normal and malignant cells, *J. Cell. Physiol.*, 99, 279, 1979.
129. Croce, C. M., Cancer genes in cell hybrids, *Biochim. Biophys. Acta*, 605, 411, 1980.
130. Weissman, B. E. and Stanbridge, E. J., Complexity of control of tumorigenic expression in intraspecies hybrids of human SV40-transformed fibroblasts and normal human fibroblasts cell lines, *Cytogenet. Cell Genet.*, 35, 263, 1983.
131. Stanbridge, E. J., Flandemeyer, R. R., Daniels, F. W., and Nelson-Rees, W. A., Specific chromosome loss associated with the expression of tumorigenicity in human cell hybrids, *Somat. Cell Genet.*, 7, 699, 1981.
132. Stoler, A. and Bouck, N., Identification of a single chromosome in the normal human genome essential for suppression of hamster cell transformation, *Proc. Natl. Acad. Sci. U.S.A.*, 82, 570, 1985.
133. Klinger, H. P. and Shows, T. B., Suppression of tumorigenicity in somatic cell hybrids: human chromosomes implicated as suppressors of tumorigenicity in hybrids with Chinese hamster ovary cells, *J. Natl. Cancer Inst.*, 71, 559, 1983.
134. Evans, E. P., Burteshaw, M. D., Brown, B. B., Hennion, R., and Harris, H., The analysis of malignancy by cell fusion, *J. Cell Sci.*, 56, 113, 1982.
135. Jonasson, J., Porey, S., and Harris, H., The analysis of malignancy by cell fusion: cytogenetic analysis of hybrids between malignant and diploid cells and of tumors derived from them, *J. Cell Sci.*, 24, 217, 1977.
136. Ziegler, M. L., Phenotypic expression of malignancy in hybrid and cybrid mouse cells, *Somat. Cell Genet.*, 4, 477, 1978.
137. Howell, A. N. and Sager, R., Tumorigenicity and its suppression in cybrids of mouse and Chinese hamster cell lines, *Proc. Natl. Acad. Sci. U.S.A.*, 75, 2358, 1978.
138. Koura, M., Isaka, H., Voshida, M. C., Tosu, M., and Sekiguehi, T., Suppression of tumorigenicity in interspecific reconstituted cells and cybrids, *Gann*, 73, 574, 1982.
139. Shay, J. W., Lorkowski, B., and Clark, M. A., Suppression of tumorigenicity in cybrids, *J. Supramol. Struct. Cell. Biochem.*, 16, 75, 1981.
140. Giguere, L. and Morais, R., On suppression of tumorigenicity in hybrid and cybrid mouse cells, *Somat. Cell Genet.*, 7, 457, 1981.
141. Reitsma, P. H., Rothberg, P. G., Astrin, S. M., Trial, J., Bar-Shavit, Z., Hall, A., Teitelbaum, S. L., and Kahn, A. J., Regulation of myc gene expression in HL-60 leukemia cells by a Vitamin D metabolite, *Nature (London)*, 306, 492, 1983.
142. Lachman, H. M. and Skoultchi, A. I., Expression of c-myc changes during differentiation of mouse erythroleukaemia cells, *Nature (London)*, 310, 592, 1984.
143. Filmus, J. and Buick, R. N., Relationship of c-myc expression to differentiation and proliferation of HL-60 cells, *Cancer Res.*, 56, 822, 1985.
144. Grosso, L. E. and Pitot, H. C., Transcriptional regulation of c-myc during chemically induced differentiation of HL-60 cultures, *Cancer Res.*, 45, 847, 1985.
145. Knight, E., Jr., Anton, E. D., Fahey, D., Friedland, B. K., and Jonak, G. J., Interferon regulates c-myc gene expression in Daudi cells at the post-transcriptional level, *Proc. Natl. Acad. Sci. U.S.A.*, 82, 1151, 1985.
146. Jonak, G. J. and Knight, E., Jr., Selective reduction of c-myc mRNA in Daudi cells by human β-interferon, *Proc. Natl. Acad. Sci. U.S.A.*, 81, 1747, 1984.
147. Croce, C. M., Erikson, J., Ar-Rushdi, A., Aden, D., and Nishikura, K., Translocated c-myc oncogene of Burkitt lymphoma is transcribed in plasma cells and repressed in lymphoblastoid cells, *Proc. Natl. Acad. Sci. U.S.A.*, 81, 3170, 1984.
148. Nishikura, K., Erickson, J., Ar-Rushdi, A., Huebner, K., and Croce, C. M., The translocated c-myc oncogene of Raji Burkitt lymphoma cells is not expressed in human lymphoblastoid cells, *Proc. Natl. Acad. Sci. U.S.A.*, 82, 2900, 1985.

gene. A well-quoted example is the methylation of a site 600 bp upstream of the chick vitellogenin gene.[40] This experiment shows that the undermethylation events can occur as a result of gene expression, and may possibly act as a cellular memory device allowing the cell to respond rapidly to subsequent hormonal signals.[41] There may therefore be two roles for methylation: one to keep genes silenced and another which occurs as the active transcription of the gene proceeds. The mechanism for the demethylation in these systems is complicated by the fact that it appears to occur in the absence of DNA synthesis and there has been only one report on the existence of demethylase enzymes.[42] It is therefore difficult to understand how the hypomethylation event could occur, since it is generally assumed to be the result of a passive process resulting from a failure to methylate during cell division. The demethylation which occurs in these systems may, however, result from a DNA repair process followed by a failure to remethylate.

These apparently contradictory results are therefore still explainable if hypomethylation is a necessary but not sufficient condition for the expression of certain but not all genes. Therefore, while there are clearly many levels of control, methylation may be considered as a primary locking device, and aberrations in this information coding system may be important in abnormal gene expression as it occurs in oncogenic transformation. The concept that changes in DNA methylation occur during neoplastic transformation and that flexibility in methylation levels and patterns are characteristic of neoplasia will therefore be examined.

IV. INHIBITION OF DNA METHYLATION BY CHEMICAL CARCINOGENS

Many experiments have suggested that ultimate chemical carcinogens, after interaction with DNA or with methyltransferase enzymes, inhibit 5-mC formation in test tube reactions and in living cells. Since Riggs and Jones[6] have recently reviewed this subject extensively, only the salient points will be re-emphasized here.

Many chemical carcinogens react preferentially with guanine residues in DNA after conversion to active electrophiles. Since guanine occurs both adjacent to and opposite to cytosine residues in CG methylation sites, the occurrence of adducts at these sites may be expected to interfere with the transfer of a methyl group from SAM to the acceptor DNA. Indeed, a large number of investigations has shown that the interaction of alkylating agents[43,44] and benzo(a)pyrene diolepoxide[45] with acceptor DNAs substantially inhibits the ability of the DNA to be modified enzymatically. These studies have not shown definitively whether it is the interaction of the carcinogen with the guanine residue at the methylation site which is important for inhibitory activity, but they establish that carcinogen-induced damage might perturb DNA methylation in living cells. The formation of single strand breaks in the DNA also lessens its ability to accept methyl groups from SAM.[45] Chemical carcinogens may therefore inhibit the methylation reaction by several different types of DNA damage.

The methyltransferase enzyme requires an active SH group for its function and interaction with MNNG directly inhibits its activity.[46] Since the amount of methyltransferase enzyme in the cell might be limited, it might be expected that interference with enzymatic function could result in hypomethylation during the S phase of the cell cycle. Chemical carcinogens may therefore inhibit methylation by at least three mechanisms, including adduct formation, formation of single strand breaks, and direct inhibition of the methyltransferase enzyme.

There is also some evidence that chemical carcinogens can decrease the DNA 5-mC content of transformable cells in culture.[45,47] However, the abilities of carcinogens to inhibit overall methylation in living cells is not seen in all cells, and we found inhibition of methylation in 3T3 but not in $10T_{1/2}$ cells exposed to benzapyrene or other carcinogens.[45,47] Alkylating agents can also inhibit methylation in tumorigenic cells[43] so that there is a clear rationale for anticipating deranged methylation patterns in cells exposed to agents which damage DNA. The net effect of this damage might be a heritable change in gene expression, and further methylation changes may occur in the cell divisions subsequent to carcinogen insult.

The advantage of the hypothesis that deranged methylation is implicated in transformation is that it does not require the continued presence of the carcinogen in DNA in order for the effects on gene expression to be manifest. It could also partly explain the fact that the frequency of oncogenic transformation is often greater than that expected for a purely mutagenic mechanism.[48] Alternatively, both mutagenic and epigenetic changes induced by carcinogens may be important in inducing alterations in structural genes, with the epigenetic component contributing to the abnormal expression of these and other genes in subsequent divisions.

V. OVERALL DNA METHYLATION LEVELS IN TRANSFORMED CELLS

A large body of experimental evidence shows that changes in overall genomic 5-mC levels occur in transformed cells.[6] These studies have demonstrated undermethylation,[49-51] no change in methylation,[52,53] and increased methylation[54] in different experimental systems. Some of these studies have utilized established cell lines as the basis of comparisons. This might present a problem in interpretation because substantial changes in DNA methylation occur when cells are explanted into tissue culture.[52] Thus, the significance of the observed changes to the tumorigenic phenotype is not entirely clear, and the studies with tumors in vivo are probably of greater significance.

The important studies of Lapeyre et al.[49,55] and Kuo et al.,[56] have indicated that hypomethylation is evident in hepatic carcinomas newly induced in rats by carcinogen treatment. However, consistent hypomethylation of the DNA in tumors freshly excised from children with a variety of neoplasias is not always observed,[53] although some tumors, particularly neuroblastomas, are significantly hypomethylated when compared to human fibroblast tissue. In a more extensive study, Ehrlich et al.,[57] and Gama-Sosa et al.,[58] observed significant undermethylation of DNA in a large series of human tumors when compared to the tissues of origin.

Overall, the results do not allow for generalizations to be made regarding DNA hypomethylation in all tumors, but are significant in suggesting that changes in DNA methylation levels can accompany oncogenic transformation. These changes may have important effects on the behavior of cells and contribute to the full development of malignant potential.

VI. METHYLATION CHANGES IN SPECIFIC GENES IN TUMORS

The relationship between decreased genomic 5-mC levels and gene expression and cell growth is not known, although it is clear that tissue-specific differences in DNA methylation level do occur. On the other hand, the relationship between hypomethylation of specific sequences within genes and their subsequent expression is more firmly established. Recent excitement therefore has been generated by experiments which have examined the methylation status of a series of genes in naturally occurring human tumors (Table 2). Feinberg and Vogelstein[59] were the first to show substantial hypomethylation of growth hormone and globin genes in primary human carcinomas. They observed hypomethylation in four out of five tumors. The use of the colon carcinoma

22. Wolf, S. F., Dintzis, S., Toniolo, D., Persico, G., Lunnen, K. D., Axelman, J., and Migeon, B. R., Complete concordance between glucose-6-phosphate dehydrogenase activity and hypomethylation of CpG clusters: implications for X-chromosome dosage compensation, *Nucleic Acids Res.*, 12, 9333, 1984.

23. Church, G. M. and Gilbert, W., Genomic sequencing, *Proc. Natl. Acad. Sci. U.S.A.*, 81, 1991, 1984.

24. Busslinger, M., Hurst, J., and Flavell, R. A., DNA methylation and the regulation of globin gene expression, *Cell*, 34, 197, 1983.

25. Langer, K.-D., Vardimon, L., Renz, D., and Doerfler, W., DNA methylation of three 5'-CCGG-3' sites in the promoter and 5' region inactivate the E2a gene of adenovirus type 2, *Proc. Natl. Acad. Sci. U.S.A.*, 81, 2950, 1984.

26. Stuhlman, H., Jahner, D., and Jaenisch, R., Infectivity and methylation of retroviral genomes is correlated with expression in the animal, *Cell*, 26, 221, 1981.

27. Gautsch, J. W. and Wilson, M. C., Delayed *de novo* methylation in teratocarcinoma suggests additional tissue specific mechanisms for controlling gene expression, *Nature (London)*, 301, 32, 1983.

28. Jove, R., Sperber, D. E., and Manley, J. L., Transcription of methylated eukaryotic viral genes in a soluble *in vitro* system, *Nucleic Acids Res.*, 12, 4715, 1984.

29. Jones, P. A. and Taylor, S. M., Cellular differentiation, cytidine analogs and DNA methylation, *Cell*, 20, 85, 1980.

30. Jones, P. A., Altering gene expression with 5-azacytidine, *Cell*, 40, 485, 1985a.

31. Jones, P. A., Effects of 5-azacytidine and its 2'-deoxyderivative on cell differentiation and DNA methylation, *Pharmac. Ther.*, 28, 17, 1985.

32. Simon, D., Stuhlman, H., Jahner, D., Wagner, H., Werner, E., and Jaenisch, R., Retrovirus genomes methylated by mammalian but not bacterial methylase are non-infectious, *Nature (London)*, 304, 275, 1983.

33. Taylor, S. M. and Jones, P. A., Mechanism of action of eukaryotic DNA methyltransferase: use of 5-azacytosine-containing DNA, *J. Mol. Biol.*, 162, 679, 1982.

34. Creusot, F., Acs, G., and Christman, J. K., Inhibition of DNA methyltransferase and induction of Friend erythroleukemia cell differentiation by 5-azacytidine and 5-aza-2'-deoxycytidine, *J. Biol. Chem.*, 257, 2041, 1982.

35. Santi, D. V., Norment, A., and Garrett, C. E., Covalent bond formation between a DNA-cytosine methyltransferase and DNA containing 5-azacytosine, *Proc. Natl. Acad. Sci. U.S.A.*, 81, 6993, 1984.

36. Venolia, L., Garther, S. M., Wassman, E. R., Yen, P., Mohandas, T., and Shapiro, L. J., Transformation with DNA from 5-azacytidine reactivated X-chromosomes, *Proc. Natl. Acad. Sci. U.S.A.*, 79, 2352, 1982.

37. McKeon, C., Chkubo, H., Pastan, I., and deCrombruggle, B., Unusual methylation pattern of the $\alpha 2(1)$ collagen gene, *Cell*, 29, 203, 1982.

38. Gerber-Huber, S., May, F. E. B., Westley, B. R., Felber, B. K., Hosbach, H. A., Andres, A.-C., and Ryffel, G. U., In contrast to other Xenopus genes the estrogen-inducible vitellogenin genes are expressed when totally methylated, *Cell*, 33, 43, 1983.

39. Cate, R. L., Chick, W., and Gilbert, W., Comparison of the methylation patterns of the two rat insulin genes, *J. Biol. Chem.*, 258, 6645, 1983.

40. Wilks, A., Seldran, M., and Jost, J. P., An estrogen-dependent demethylation at the 5' end of the chicked vitellogenin gene is independent of DNA synthesis, *Nucleic Acids Res.*, 12, 1163, 1984.

41. Bird, A. P., DNA methylation — how important is gene control?, *Nature (London)*, 307, 503, 1984.

42. Gjerset, R. A. and Martin, D. W., Presence of a DNA demethylating activity in the nucleus of murine erythroleukemia cells, *J. Biol. Chem.*, 257, 8581, 1982.

43. Boehm, T. L. J. and Drahovsky, D., Hypomethylation of DNA in Raji cells after treatment with N-methyl-N-nitrosourea, *Carcinogenesis*, 2, 39, 1981.

44. Pfohl-Leszkowicz, A., Fuchs, R. P. P., Keith, G., and Dirheimer, G., Enzymatic methylation of chicken erythrocyte DNA modified by two carcinogens 2-(N-Acetoxyacetylamino)fluorene and methyl-nitrosourea, *J. Cancer Res. Clin. Oncol.*, 103, 318, 1982.

45. Wilson, V. L. and Jones, P. A., Inhibition of DNA methylation by chemical carcinogens, *Cell*, 32, 239, 1983.

46. Cox, R., DNA methylase assay inhibition *in vitro* by N-Methyl-N'-nitro-N-nitrosoguaindine, *Cancer Res.*, 40, 61, 1980.

47. Wilson, V. L. and Jones, P. A., Chemical carcinogen-mediated decreases in DNA 5-methylcytosine content of BALB/3T3 cells, *Carcinogenesis*, 5, 1027, 1984.

48. Holliday, R., A new theory of carcinogenesis, *Br. J. Cancer*, 40, 513, 1979.

49. Lapeyre, J.-N., Walker, M. S., and Becker, F. F., DNA methylation and methylase levels in normal and malignant mouse hepatic tissues, *Carcinogenesis*, 2, 873, 1981.

50. Diala, E. S., Cheah, M. S. C., Rowitch, D., and Hoffman, R. M., Extent of DNA methylation in human tumor cells, *J. Natl. Cancer Inst.*, 71, 755, 1983.

51. Gama-Sosa, M. A., Slagel, V. A., Trewyn, R. W., Oxenhandler, R., Kuo, K., Gehrke, W., and Ehrlich, M., The 5-methylcytosine content of DNA from human tumors, *Nucleic Acids Res.*, 11, 6883, 1983.

52. Wilson, V. L. and Jones, P. A., DNA methylation decreases in aging but not in immortal cells, *Science,* 220, 1055, 1983b.

53. Flatau, E., Bogenmann, E., and Jones, P. A., Variable 5-methylcytosine levels in human tumor cell lines and fresh pediatric tumor explant, *Cancer Res.,* 43, 4901, 1983.

54. Gunthert, V., Schweiger, M., Stupp, M., and Doerfler, W., DNA methylation in adenovirus, adenovirus-transformed cells, and host cells, *Proc. Natl. Acad. Sci. U.S.A.,* 73, 3923, 1976.

55. Lapeyre, J.-N. and Becker, F. F., 5-methylcytosine content of nuclear DNA during chemical hepatocarcinogenesis and in carcinomas which result, *Biochem. Biophys. Res. Commun.,* 87, 698, 1979.

56. Kuo, M. T., Iyer, B., Wu, J. R., Lapeyre, J.-N., and Becker, F. F., Methylation of the α-fetoprotein gene in productive and nonproductive rat hepatocellular carcinomas, *Cancer Res.,* 44, 1642, 1984.

57. Ehrlich, M., Gama-Sosa, M. A., Huang, L.-H., Midgett, R. M., Kuo, K. C., McCune, R. A., and Gehrke, C., Amount and distribution of 5-methylcytosine in human DNA from different types of tissues or cells, *Nucleic Acids Res.,* 10, 2709, 1982.

58. Gama-Sosa, M. A., Midgett, R. M., Slagel, V. A., Githens, S., Kuo, K. C., Gehrke, C. W., and Ehrlich, M., Tissue specific differences in DNA methylation in various mammals, *Biochim. Biophys. Acta,* 740, 212, 1983.

59. Feinberg, A. P. and Vogelstein, B., Hypomethylation distinguishes genes of some human cancers from their normal counterparts, *Nature (London),* 301, 89, 1983.

60. Feinberg, A. P. and Vogelstein, B., Hypomethylation of ras oncogenes in primary human cancers, *Biochem. Biophys. Res. Commun.,* 111, 47, 1983.

61. Goelz, S. E., Vogelstein, B., Hamilton, S. R., and Feinberg, A. P., DNA from benign and malignant human colon neoplasms is hypomethylated, *Science,* 228, 187, 1985.

62. Mays-Hoopes, L., Brown, A., and Huang, R. C. C., Methylation and rearrangement of mouse intracisternal A particle genes in development, aging and myeloma, *Mol. Cell. Biol.,* 3, 1371, 1983.

63. Morgan, R. A. and Huang, R. C. C., Correlation of undermethylation of intracisternal A-particle genes with expression in murine plasmacytomas but not in NIH/3T3 embryo fibroblasts, *Cancer Res.,* 44, 5234, 1984.

64. Benedict, W. F., Banerjee, A., Gardner, A., and Jones, P. A., Induction of morphological transformation in mouse C3H/10T$_{1/2}$ clone 8 cells and chromosomal damage in hamster A(T$_1$)Cl-3 cells by cancer chemotherapeutic agents, *Cancer Res.,* 37, 2202, 1977.

65. Harrison, J. J., Anisowicz, A., Gadi, I. K., Raffeld, M., and Sager, R., Azacytidine-induced tumorigenesis of CHEF/18 cells: correlated DNA methylation and chromosome changes, *Proc. Natl. Acad. Sci. U.S.A.,* 80, 6606, 1983.

66. Bouck, N., Kokkinakis, D., and Ostrowsky, J., Induction of a step in carcinogenesis that is normally associated with mutagenesis by nonmutagenic concentrations of 5-azacytidine, *Mol. Cell. Biol.,* 4, 1231, 1984.

67. Landolph, J. R. and Jones, P. A., Mutagenicity of 5-azacytidine and related nucleosides in C3H/10T$_{1/2}$ C18 and V79 cells, *Cancer Res.,* 42, 817, 1982.

68. Frost, P., Liteplo, R. G., Donaghue, R. P., and Kerbel, R. S., The selection of strongly immunogenic "Tum-" variants from tumors at high frequency using 5-azacytidine, *J. Exp. Med.,* 159, 1491, 1984.

69. Stoner, G. D., Shimkin, M. B., Kniazeff, A. J., Weisburger, J. H., Weisburger, E. K., and Gori, G. B., Test for carcinogenicity of food additives and chemotherapeutic agents by pulmonary tumor response in strain A mice, *Cancer Res.,* 33, 3069, 1973.

70. Carr, B. I., Reilly, J. G., Smith, S. S., Winberg, C., and Riggs, A., The tumorigenicity of 5-azacytidine in the male Fischer rat, *Carcinogenesis,* 5, 1583, 1984.

71. Dendra, A., Rao, P. M., Rajalakshmi, S., and Sarma, D. S. R., 5-Azacytidine potentiates initiation induced by carcinogens in the rat liver, *Carcinogenesis,* 6, 145, 1985.

72. Kerbel, R. S., Frost, P., Liteplo, R., Carlow, D., and Elliot, B. E., Possible epigenetic mechanisms of tumor progression: induction of high frequency heritable but phenotypically unstable changes in the tumorigenic and metastatic properties of tumor cell populations by 5-azacytidine treatment, *J. Cell. Physiol. Suppl.,* 3, 87, 1984.

73. Olsson, L. and Forchhammer, J., Induction of the metastatic phenotype in a mouse tumor model by 5-azacytidine, and characterization of an antigen associated with metastatic activity, *Proc. Natl. Acad. Sci. U.S.A.,* 81, 3389, 1984.

74. Hancock, M. C. and Smith, H. S., Phenotypic variability in anchorage-independent growth by a human breast tumor cell line, *J. Natl. Cancer Inst.,* 72, 833, 1984.

75. Olsson, L., Due, C., and Diamont, M., Treatment of human cell lines with 5-azacytidine may result in profound alterations in clonogenicity and growth rate, *J. Cell Biol.,* 100, 508, 1985.

76. Olsson, L., Behnke, O., and Sorensen, H. R., Modulatory effects of 5-azacytidine, phorbol ester and retinoic acid on the malignant phenotype of human lung cancer cells, *Int. J. Cancer,* 35, 189, 1985.
77. Taylor, S. M. and Jones, P. A., Multiple new phenotypes induced in $10T_{1/2}$ and 3T3 cells treated with 5-azacytidine, *Cell,* 17, 771, 1979.
78. Bodner, A. J., Ting, R. C., and Gallo, R. C., Induction of differentiation of human promyelocytic leukemia cells (HL-60) by nucleosides and methotrexate, *J. Natl. Cancer Inst.,* 67, 1025, 1981.
79. Christman, J. K., Mendelsohn, N., Herzog, D., and Schneiderman, N., Effect of 5-azacytidine on differentiation and DNA methylation in human promyelocytic leukemia cells (HL-60), *Cancer Res.,* 43, 763, 1983.
80. Faille, A., Turmel, P., and Charron, D. J., Differentiated expression of HLA-DR and HLA-DC/DS molecules in a patient with hairy cell leukemia: restoration of HLA-DC/DS expression by TPA, 5-azacytidine and sodium butyrate, *Blood,* 64, 33, 1984.
81. Pinto, A., Attadia, V., Fusco, A., Ferrara, F., Spada, O. A., and DiFiore, P., 5-aza-2'-deoxycytidine induces terminal differentiation of leukemic blasts from patients with acute myeloid leukemias, *Blood,* 64, 992, 1984.
82. Chiu, C.-P. and Blau, H. M., 5-Azacytidine permits gene activation in a previously non-inducible cell type, *Cell,* 40, 417, 1985.

Chapter 3

SUPPRESSION OF TUMORIGENICITY IN MAMMALIAN CELL HYBRIDS

Bernard E. Weissman

TABLE OF CONTENTS

I. INTRODUCTION

The molecular basis of cancer has been the subject of intense investigation over the past several decades. Although the many facets of cellular transformation have been well-documented, the event(s) which is responsible for these changes has yet to be determined. In order to investigate the processes of malignant transformation, several models of cancer have been developed, including transformation of cells both in vitro and in the animal by both chemical carcinogens and oncogenic viruses. However, some of the most interesting studies have involved the use of somatic cell hybrids formed between tumorigenic cells and their normal counterparts.

Somatic cell hybrids between two cells were first isolated as a spontaneous event in cell culture by Barski et al.[1] in 1960. These cell hybrids were produced by coculturing the two parental cell types together for an extended period. The identification of the hybrid cells was due to their overgrow of one of the parental cell populations. However, viable hybrid cell formation turned out to be a relatively rare event in tissue culture. This led to refinements of somatic cell hybridization techniques, including the development of selective media for hybrid cells as well as the use of fusogens to increase the formation of these cells.[2-5]

These improved procedures for the isolation of somatic cell hybrids have led to a variety of studies aimed at determining the genetic behavior of tumorigenicity. For the purposes of this chapter, tumorigenicity is defined as the ability of a cell to form a progressively growing tumor in an appropriate host animal, usually a newborn syngeneic or an immunosuppressed mouse. The ability of a cell to metastasize in the animal will not be considered, as genetic studies on the behavior of this parameter are still in progress. At this time, the majority of studies based on somatic cell hybrids between tumorigenic and normal cells supports the concept that tumorigenicity behaves as a recessive genetic trait. These studies have been reviewed recently and will be mentioned only in an historical light.[6,7] The focus of this review will be on what new information has been gained from a study of these somatic cell hybrids both in vivo and in vitro, and what these results imply about the process of malignant transformation in human cells.

II. TUMORIGENIC EXPRESSION IN CELL HYBRIDS

In 1960, Barski et al.[1,8,9] first examined the genetic behavior of tumorigenicity in somatic cell hybrids between a highly tumorigenic cell line, NCTC 2472, and a poorly tumorigenic cell line, NCTC 2555. Their studies showed that the hybrid cells were as tumorigenic as the parental NCTC 2472 cells. Their conclusion was that tumorigenicity appeared to act as a dominant genetic trait in this system. Following these initial studies, several other investigators confirmed these findings using a variety of other cell lines as the tumorigenic parent, including polyoma-transformed mouse fibroblasts and mouse melanoma cells. By the end of the decade, the evidence from a number of laboratories was that tumorigenicity behaved as a dominant genetic trait (Table 1).

Despite the evidence from these previous studies, Harris and co-workers[10] decided to re-evaluate the data with an emphasis on the chromosomal complements of both the parental and hybrid populations. The results of their investigations on hybrid cells formed between different highly tumorigenic mouse cell lines and an L cell line of low tumorigenic potential were that suppression of tumorigenicity was observed when the hybrid cells retained the full chromosomal complement of both parental cells. Tumors formed by the hybrid cells were invariably shown to have lost a large number of chromosomes when compared to the preinjection cell lines.[10,11] These results were later

Table 1
STUDIES USING INTRASPECIFIC MOUSE CELL HYBRIDS

Year	Tumorigenic parental cell	Nontumorigenic or low tumorigenic parental cell	Ref.
	Tumorigenicity is dominant		
1961	NCTC 2472-fibrosarcoma	NCTC 2555-fibroblasts	1, 8
1965	NCTC 2472	Normal fibroblasts	75
1967	Py27-polyoma-transformed fibro-blasts	Normal fibroblasts	76
	B6-melanoma	A9-L cell derivative; fibroblasts	77
1970	B6	A9	78
1976	PCCazal-teratocarcinoma	Normal thymocytes	21
1977	Cl-1D-fibrosarcoma	Normal lymphocytes	79
	Cl-1D	Normal mouse cells in vivo	80
1980	Cloudman S-91-melanoma	Normal mouse cells in vivo	81
	Cloudman PBL-22-melanoma	Embryo fibroblasts	81
	Tumorigenicity is recessive		
1969	Ehrlich-mammary carcinoma	A9	10
	SEWA-polyoma-transformed fi-broblast	A9	10
1971	YAC-lymphoma	A9	11
	MSWBS-ascites sarcoma	A9	11
	Ehrlich	Normal fibroblasts	82
	TA$_3$-mammary adenocarcinoma	Normal fibroblasts	83
1977	MEL 2C-melanoma	Normal fibroblasts	63
	PG-19-melanoma	Normal fibroblasts	63
	YACIR-lymphoma	Normal fibroblasts	63
	SEWA	Normal fibroblasts	63
	A9HT-fibrosarcoma	Normal fibroblasts	84

extended to include hybrid cell lines derived from tumorigenic mouse cells and normal diploid mouse fibroblasts (Table 1). Thus, Harris and co-workers concluded that tumorigenicity behaved as a recessive genetic trait in somatic cell hybrids and that re-expression of tumorigenic potential was correlated with a loss of chromosomes from the cells. Studies from other laboratories have confirmed these results as summarized in Table 1.

Since these early studies on mouse intraspecific cell hybrids, many investigators have used cells from other species to study the genetics of tumorigenic expression in mammalian cells. These species have included intraspecific cell hybrids of Chinese hamster cells or human cell lines, as well as interspecific cell hybrids between different rodent species or rodent and human cell lines. Each system has its relative merits and has provided valuable information about the control of tumorigenic expression in mammalian cells. A review of these studies supports the concept that tumorigenicity behaves as a recessive genetic trait.

In the early 1970s, Berebbi and Barski[12] produced hybrid cells between a highly tumorigenic Chinese hamster cell and a sister cell line which was nontumorigenic in cortisone-treated hamsters. The hybrid cells displayed a range of tumorigenic potentials from completely suppressed to highly tumorigenic. Interestingly, there were no major differences in the total chromosome number between any of the hybrid cells.

More recently, Sager and Kovac[13] have developed a pair of isogenic, pseudodiploid Chinese hamster cell lines which have proved useful for somatic cell hybrid studies.

Table 2

STUDIES USING HUMAN INTRASPECIFIC HYBRID CELLS

Year	Tumorigenic parental cell	Nontumorigenic parental cell	Ref.
1976	D98-HeLa derivative; cervical carcinoma	Normal fibroblasts	14
1980	D98	Normal fibroblasts	39
1982	HeLa	Normal fibroblasts	40
	D98	Normal keratinocytes	85
1985	D98	Normal smooth muscle	86
	D98	Normal endothelial	87
1984	HT1080-fibrosarcoma	Normal fibroblasts	57
1985	EJ-bladder carcinoma	Normal fibroblasts	59
	A549-lung carcinoma	Normal fibroblasts	87
	A673-rhabdomyosarcoma	Normal fibroblasts	86

One cell line, designated CHEF/18, was nontumorigenic, required high serum for growth, and failed to proliferate in semisolid medium. The other cell line, CHEF/16, was highly tumorigenic, grew in low serum, and was anchorage-independent. Hybrids between these two cell lines were suppressed for tumorigenic potential, supporting the concept that tumorigenicity behaved as a recessive genetic trait in Chinese hamster cells.

The human intraspecific cell hybrid system has also been useful for the study of the control of expression of tumorigenicity. Initial studies by Stanbridge[14] in 1976 demonstrated that cell hybrids formed between HeLa, (a cervical carcinoma cell line) and normal human fibroblasts were absolutely suppressed for tumorigenic potential. Since these initial studies, the suppression of tumorigenicity in human cell hybrids has been shown to be a generalized phenomenon. As shown in Table 2, a variety of normal cells from different human tissues is capable of suppressing the tumorigenic potential of the HeLa cell line. Furthermore, the tumorigenicity of cell lines which are derived from both mesenchymal and ectodermal tissue are also suppressed when hybridized to normal human fibroblasts. These data clearly establish the recessive genetic behavior of tumorigenicity in human cells. The only exception to these results was studies by Croce et al.[15] showing that hybrids between a human fibrosarcoma and normal human fibroblasts were tumorigenic. However, a more recent study has demonstrated suppression of tumorigenicity in that system.

Many investigators have used rodent-rodent or rodent-human interspecific cell hybrids due to the difficulty of identifying the parental origin of chromosomes in intraspecific cell hybrids. Cell hybrids formed between two different species preferentially lose chromosomes of one of the parental species. With the development of chromosome banding techniques for the identification of individual chromosomes, investigators could potentially determine specific chromosomes associated with the suppression of tumorigenic potential. However, studies on the expression of tumorigenic potential in interspecific hybrid cells have often given conflicting results, as summarized in Table 3. There have been reports of both complete suppression and complete lack of suppression in interspecific rodent cells. Again the majority of the results supports the recessive nature of tumorigenic potential, but the data are not always clear.

The studies of Jonasson and Harris,[12] and those of Kucherlapati and Shin,[16] can be reconciled perhaps by closer examination of the data. The former group reported that hybrid cells formed between PG-19 and normal human fibroblasts were suppressed in their ability to form tumors in nude mice. However, a later report from the second group stated that tumorigenicity behaved as a dominant trait in hybrid cells formed

Table 3
STUDIES USING INTERSPECIFIC HYBRID CELLS

Year	Tumorigenic parental cell	Nontumorigenic or poorly tumorigenic parental cell	Ref.
	Tumorigenicity is dominant		
1973	R4/B-mouse fibrosarcoma	D/AD/Aza-Chinese hamster fibroblasts	88
1979	A9-mouse fibrosarcoma	Normal human fibroblasts	16
	PG-19-mouse melanoma	Normal human fibroblasts	16
	HT1080-human fibrosarcoma	Normal mouse fibroblasts	15
1981	Wg3-h-o-Chinese hamster fibrosarcoma	Normal mouse fibroblasts	89
	Tumorigenicity is recessive		
1976	RAG-mouse	Normal human fibroblasts	90
1977	PG-19	Normal human lymphocytes	17
	PG-19	Normal human fibroblasts	17
1978	TA3B-mouse mammary carcinoma	Rat embryo fibroblasts	28
	PG-19	Normal human lymphocytes	91
	PG-19	Normal human fibroblasts	91
	A9	Normal human fibroblasts	92
	CHO-Chinese hamster fibrosarcoma	Normal human fibroblasts	92
1979	DC3F-Chinese hamster fibrosarcoma	Mouse 3T3 fibroblasts	7
	A549-human lung carcinoma	Mouse 3T3 fibroblasts	34
1981	PG-19	Normal human lymphocytes	93
	DON-Chinese hamster fibrosarcoma	Normal human lymphocytes	93

between PG-19 cells and different normal human fibroblasts. The conclusions drawn by Kucherlapati and Shin were based on two observations: one was that all of the hybrid cells were capable of forming tumors; and second, all human chromosomes were represented at least once in the tumors derived from the hybrid cells. However, the data were also consistent with the previous reports from Harris' group in that (1) there was a reduced take incidence for the hybrid cells, and (2) the total chromosome complement was markedly reduced in the tumor cells as compared to the original hybrid cells. Furthermore, Evans et al.[18] raise the point that the presence of all human chromosomes in at least one of the tumor cells is unimportant if gene dosage plays a role in the expression of tumorigenicity. A second caveat that one has to deal with in interspecific hybrid cells is the expression of foreign DNA in a different genetic background. The data in the report of Kucherlapati and Shin clearly showed that while some human chromosomes were present by banding techniques, there was no detectable expression of genes present on those chromosomes. These two reports illustrate some of the pitfalls one can encounter in interpreting data from somatic cell hybrid studies.

Although tumorigenicity appears to behave as a recessive genetic trait in most systems, there are two clear exceptions. These are in systems where either lymphoid cells or virally-transformed cells are studied. In the case of lymphoid cells, hybrid cells formed between myeloma and normal bone marrow cells result in the formation of the well-characterized hybridoma cell lines.[19] Injection of hybridoma cells into an appropriate animal results in tumor formation. Chromosome analyses have shown that the loss of chromosomes from the hybrid cells apparently does not play a role in these results.[19] Jonasson and Harris[17] have also shown that normal human lymphoid cells are not as efficient in suppressing the tumorigenic potential of mouse tumor cell lines as normal human fibroblasts. In other studies, Weissman and Stanbridge[20] have demonstrated that human cell hybrids using tumorigenic lymphoid cells as one parent were not suppressed for tumorigenicity, where other types of human tumors were. Miller and Ruddle[21] have reported that hybrid cells between a mouse teratocarcinoma cell line and normal mouse thymocytes are tumorigenic when assayed in nude mice. These results may indicate that cells from the lymphoid system, which are normally capable of dividing throughout the lifetime of the animal, are under a different type of growth control than other types of nondividing normal tissue. Indeed, while normal human fibroblasts invariably become senescent in culture, lymphoid cells appear to develop easily into permanent cell lines. These findings raise obvious questions about differences in the etiologies of human leukemias and lymphomas, and those of carcinomas, sarcomas, etc.

In studies where virally-transformed cell lines are involved, the picture is less clear. Several investigators have reported that the behavior of tumorigenicity in hybrids between either SV_{40}-transformed- or polyoma-transformed cell lines and normal fibroblasts is no different than in cases involving spontaneously or chemically transformed tumorigenic cell lines.[17,22,23] However, Koprowski and Croce[24] have demonstrated that hybrid cells formed between SV_{40}-transformed human fibroblasts and normal mouse peritoneal macrophages were highly tumorigenic. Weissman and Stanbridge[25] have shown that in hybrids between SV_{40}-transformed human fibroblasts and normal human fibroblasts, a range of tumorigenicity was observed from completely suppressed to highly tumorigenic. One case was observed where a nontumorigenic clone of the SV_{40}-transformed cell line fused to a normal human fibroblast resulted in a tumorigenic hybrid cell. In studies involving retrovirus-transformed cells, the results were similar.[26] Some investigators have shown suppression of tumorigenicity in appropriate cell hybrids, while others have observed expression of tumorigenicity. It is therefore difficult to come to a conclusion about the genetic behavior of tumorigenicity in virally transformed cells. This is not surprising considering that virally-transformed cells have incorporated exogenous genetic information in their genomes. There is also the added complication of different levels of viral gene products in different cells as well as the instability of the integration site of the viral genome. All of these parameters have made the interpretation of the results from these studies difficult. It is apparent that in some cases tumorigenic potential can be suppressed in virally-transformed cells. Whether this is accomplished by the same mechanisms involved in the suppression of other types of tumor cells remains to be seen.

An intriguing possibility raised by the suppression of tumorigenicity in cell hybrids between tumorigenic and normal cells is that of complementation between different tumorigenic cell lines. Thus if more than one genetic defect is involved in the expression of tumorigenicity, two cell lines with different defects may be able to complement each other, resulting in a cell hybrid suppressed for tumorigenicity. When Wiener and co-workers[27] investigated this possibility in the mouse intraspecific hybrid system, they found only one case of apparent complementation in crosses involving 12 different tumorigenic cell lines. This was characterized by a reduction in take incidence from 100 to 67%.

More dramatic evidence has been obtained by other investigators in the field. Marshall and Dave[28] have shown the suppression of tumorigenicity as measured by take incidence in cell hybrids between mouse mammary tumor cells and Syrian hamster sarcoma cells. Geurts van Kessel et al.[29] have reported a decreased take incidence for hybrid cells between a Chinese hamster fibroblast cell line and an Rauscher Leukemia Virus (RLV)-induced mouse myeloid cell line. Weissman and Stanbridge[20] have shown complete suppression of tumorigenic potential for hybrid cells derived from human tumor cell lines of different developmental lineage. Choi et al.[30] also reported that hybrids between two SV_{40}-transformed human fibroblasts and HeLa cells were totally suppressed for tumorigenicity. This is similar to the suppression in hybrids between PG-19 and tumorigenic SV_{40}-transformed mouse fibroblasts observed by Gee and Harris.[22] Thus it appears that at least two complementation groups for the control of expression of tumorigenicity in mammalian cells exist and that they both appear to act in a recessive genetic manner.

III. THE TRANSFORMED PHENOTYPE OF CELL HYBRIDS

The study of both normal and tumorigenic cells in culture has led to the description of many parameters in vitro which correlate with tumorigenic potential in vivo. These features can be grouped together under the heading of the transformed phenotype of cells in culture. Included in this group are changes such as anchorage-independent growth, growth in low serum concentrations, loss of contact inhibition, and changes in cell-surface proteins. Attempts to correlate these changes with tumorigenicity have often been hampered by the difficulty of distinguishing between changes due to malignant transformation and alterations due to growth in tissue culture.

The availability of somatic cell hybrids between tumorigenic and normal cells has provided a test system for in vitro correlates to tumorigenicity. In many systems, it has been possible to isolate matched sets of hybrid cells which differ only by their ability to form tumors in an appropriate animal. Thus, a true in vitro marker for tumorigenicity will only be expressed by the tumorigenic parental and hybrid cells, and not by the nontumorigenic parental and hybrid cells. Analyses of these hybrid systems have led to the identification of new markers for tumorigenicity as well as ruling out other established markers as absolute correlates.

The rodent intraspecific and interspecific hybrid system has been studied extensively for in vitro parameters which might be correlated to tumorigenicity in vivo. Straus et al.[31] examined several growth parameters of mouse intraspecific cell hybrids which had been suggested as good in vitro markers for tumorigenicity. They reported no correlation with tumorigenicity for serum requirement, cloning efficiency in soft agarose, density-dependent inhibition of growth, and secretion of plasminogen activator in their mouse intraspecific hybrid cells. Sager's group[13,32] has also shown in several studies that tumorigenicity, anchorage-independent growth, and low serum requirement are all initially suppressed in hybrid cells between the tumorigenic CHEF/16 and the normal CHEF/18 cell lines. However, all three parameters can be shown to independently segregate of one another after chromosome loss.[32] Thus, it appears that more than one gene controls these growth parameters. Similar results have been reported by Marshall and Dave[28,33] for hybrids between tumorigenic mouse cells and normal rat fibroblasts. In hybrid cells between a human lung carcinoma and 3T3 cells, growth in agarose and tumor-forming ability were also discordantly expressed.[34]

One change which has correlated in the mouse intraspecific cell hybrid system has been alterations in hexose transport. The initial findings showed that there was differential binding of two lectins between tumorigenic and nontumorigenic hybrids. A protein of a molecular weight of approximately 100K was identified which bound the lectin wheat germ agglutinin in normal parental cells and nontumorigenic hybrid cells, but bound concanavalin A in tumorigenic parental and hybrid cells.[35] White and co-workers[36] later showed that this protein played a role in hexose transport into cells. Furthermore, they have linked a decrease in the Michaelis constant of hexose uptake with the tumorigenic potential of a cell.[37] Whether this decrease is directly involved in the process of cellular transformation has not been determined.

In the human intraspecific cell hybrid system, the results from several laboratories have been remarkably consistent. In general, nontumorigenic hybrids between HeLa and a variety of normal human fibroblasts display all of the transformed phenotypes usually associated with tumorigenicity.[38 40] These include expression of fibronectin, growth in low serum, secretion of plasminogen activator, and growth in semisolid medium. Upon re-expression of tumorigenicity in the hybrid cells, the majority of these parameters remains unaltered.[38,41,42] These results clearly establish that in human cells, the transformed phenotype and tumorigenic potential are under separate genetic controls.

An alternative approach is to use hybrid cells to identify new markers of transformation in vitro. In the human hybrid system, this was accomplished by raising antisera to both the tumorigenic and nontumorigenic hybrid cells in appropriate animals. Using the nontumorigenic hybrid cells to absorb out common antigens from the antiserum raised against the tumorigenic hybrid, Der and Stanbridge[43] identified a 75-kdaltons glycophosphoprotein which appeared on the surface of the tumorigenic parental and hybrid cells. The presence of this protein absolutely correlated with tumorigenic potential in the HeLa X normal human fibroblast hybrid cells. Examination of other pairs of tumorigenic and nontumorigenic human hybrid cells may identify proteins which have potential uses for diagnostic and chemotherapeutic protocols.

A final note on this subject is the question of immortality in human cells. Normal human cells from a variety of tissues display a limited lifespan in culture. There are several reports in the literature now where this limited cell growth appears to behave as a dominant genetic trait in hybrids between normal human cells and tumorigenic cell lines.[40,44,45] If this is the case, then the implication is that a third gene is involved in the process of malignant transformation — one that allows a cell to escape from cellular senescence. A second line of evidence supporting this concept is the demonstration of mutagen-treated normal human fibroblasts which are anchorage independent yet still become senescent.[46] Further studies need to be carried out in order to identify the number of genes involved in the control of the transformed phenotype in somatic cell hybrids.

IV. ONCOGENE EXPRESSION IN HYBRID CELLS

The degree of involvement of oncogenes in the process of malignant transformation has not been clearly defined. Several decades ago, many investigators felt that retroviruses which carried these dominant-acting transforming genes played a primary role in the etiology of human cancer. Indeed, many acute transforming retroviruses can cause tumors upon injection into a variety of species. In humans, however, only the family of the HTLV retroviruses appears to be causally involved in human malignancies. Thus it is unlikely that retroviruses are involved in the formation of most human cancers.

Interest has been renewed in the prospects of oncogene involvement in human cancer by the discovery of activated oncogenes in human tumor cell lines. The oncogenes present in retroviruses presumably arose by recombination between RNA leukemia viruses and genes in the vertebrate genome known as proto-oncogenes. Proto-oncogenes isolated from a variety of species do not appear to transform mouse fibroblasts in culture under physiological conditions. However, proto-oncogenes from some human tumor cell lines have become structurally altered and are now capable of transforming these mouse fibroblasts in vitro. These have included members of the *ras* oncogene family as well as some previously unidentified oncogenes such as *B-lym* and *neu.*[47-52] Furthermore, other known oncogenes, while structurally unaltered, are expressed at abnormally high levels in other human tumors.[53-55] These findings again raise the question of whether these genes contribute to the process of malignant transformation in mammalian cells.

Surprisingly, little information has been reported about the expression of these oncogenes in cell hybrid studies. In the human intraspecific hybrid cell system, two cell lines which have activated *ras* genes have been fused to normal human fibroblasts. The first study involved HT 1080, a fibrosarcoma which has an activated *N-ras* gene.[56] These hybrid cells were totally suppressed for tumorigenic potential, yet preliminary evidence showed that there was continued expression of the p21 protein, the product of the *ras* oncogene family.[57,58] Similar results were also observed in hybrids between the EJ bladder carcinoma cell line, which contains an activated *H-ras*, and normal human fibroblasts.[47] The induction of high levels of the p21 protein in the suppressed hybrids by DNA transfection of an activated *H-ras* oncogene was not sufficient for expression of tumorigenicity in the cells.[59] Therefore, the addition of normal genetic information to these tumor cells resulted in a suppression of tumorigenic potential without a concomitant reduction in the expression of the p21 protein.

The difference in action of the *ras* oncogene family in mouse fibroblasts vs. human intraspecific hybrid cells is not surprising. In the first case, the genes are being transferred to a new genetic environment in which normal regulatory controls may not be functional across species. Furthermore, the location of control elements for the *ras* oncogene family is unknown and may not be cotransferred with the structural genes. Examples of this phenomenon already exist in the case of globin gene expression. Globin gene products may be expressed in mouse fibroblast by DNA transfection, yet extinction of their expression occurs in hybrid cells between erythrocytes and mouse fibroblasts.[60,61]

The involvement of other oncogenes, such as *c-myc*, *N-myc*, *sis*, and *abl*, (which have been shown to be overexpressed in human tumors in cellular transformation and tumorigenicity), is unknown at this time. More investigations using somatic cell hybrids may provide useful information on this subject. Indeed, it would be particularly interesting to examine some of the questions in the rodent intraspecific hybrid cell system, where suppression of both tumorigenicity and transformation is observed. These genes may play a role in controlling the expression of the transformed phenotype. Alternatively, it may be intriguing to examine the expression of the *myc* oncogene family on human intraspecific hybrid cells which have a limited lifespan. The *myc* oncogene family has been implicated as an "immortalizing" agent for rodent cells.[62]

V. CHARACTERIZATION OF RECESSIVE CANCER GENES

The majority of evidence from somatic cell hybridization studies is that the addition of normal genetic information to tumor cell lines from a variety of species leads to a suppression of tumorigenicity. The implication from these studies is that there are genes in the mammalian genome which act in a recessive manner in the process of malignant transformation. In this section, I plan to discuss some of the information that is currently available about where these genes reside and what role they might play in normal cells.

Most hybrid cells between tumorigenic and nontumorigenic cells will be suppressed for tumor-forming ability. Upon continued passage in culture, variant cells will appear which have regained their tumorigenic potential, often having a reduced number of chromosomes. Harris and his co-workers,[18,63] examined a series of hybrids between different mouse tumor cell lines and normal mouse fibroblasts in hopes of determining whether any specific chromosomes were lost upon re-expression of tumorigenicity. They reported that only one mouse chromosome appeared to be lost consistently from the nontumorigenic hybrid cells upon re-expression of tumorigenic potential — chromosome 4. More importantly, by using polymorphisms of the centromeric heterochromatin, Evans et al.[18] showed that the copies of chromosome 4 that were lost from the hybrids came from the normal fibroblast parent. Further studies have located the region that is important for suppression to the lower part of the upper half of chromosome 4;[63] however, formal proof that the normal chromosome 4 carries sufficient genetic information to suppress tumorigenicity must still be performed.

Marshall[64] examined the chromosomes involved in the control of the transformed phenotype in the Chinese hamster intraspecific hybrid cell system. Detailed karotypic analyses showed that suppression of the ability to grow in soft agar correlated with the presence of the normal chromosome 1. In a related set of experiments, Harrison et al.[65] demonstrated that in chemically transformed CHEF/18 cell lines, tumorigenicity was correlated with the presence of an extra copy of chromosome 3. However, the role of this chromosome in the control of expression of tumorigenicity in the Chinese hamster cell hybrid system has not been investigated.

Klinger and Shows[66] have studied the ability of different human chromosomes to suppress the tumorigenicity of a Chinese hamster cell line. Hybrid cells between hamster and human cells preferentially lose human chromosomes upon continued passage in culture. They studied a large number of tumorigenic and nontumorigenic hybrid cells between a tumorigenic Chinese hamster cell line and normal human fibroblasts, as well as tumor cell lines derived from the hybrids. No chromosome was found that absolutely correlated with tumorigenic potential in this system. However, chromosomes 9, 10, 11, and 17 were correlated with reduced tumorigenic potential in these cells, and chromosome 2 was not observed in any of the tumor cell lines.[66] The investigators also performed a pairwise analysis to determine whether two chromosomes together were associated with suppression of tumorigenicity. Their findings implicated combinations which included chromosomes 4, 7, 8, 9, 10, 11, 13, and 17 as being involved in suppression.[66]

Stanbridge et al.[67] examined matched pairs of HeLa X normal human fibroblast hybrid cells in which one cell was nontumorigenic while the sister cell line was tumorigenic. An analysis of the chromosomal contents of these cells revealed that a reduction in the total number of chromosomes 11 and 14 was associated with re-expression of tumorigenicity in the hybrid cells. In a second set of experiments, Benedict et al.[57] demonstrated that loss of chromosomes 1 and 4 was correlated with the expression of tumorigenicity in human fibrosarcoma by normal fibroblast hybrid cells. Thus it appeared that different chromosomes were involved in the suppression of tumorigenicity in different human cells. These results would lend support to the concept that at least two genes are involved in the control of the expression of tumorigenic potential. (Hybrid cells between HeLa and this same fibrosarcoma are also suppressed for tumorigenicity.)

The initial studies in human intraspecific hybrid cells were unable to distinguish the parental origin of the chromosomes that were lost from the hybrids upon re-expression of tumorigenicity. However, with the development of restriction fragment length polymorphisms (RFLPs), one can now determine the identity of each member of homologous chromosome pairs in cells. By utilizing RFLP differences to distinguish each chromosome 11 in HeLa X fibroblast hybrids, Srivatsan et al.[68] have been able to show that the chromosome 11s from the normal parent are absent in the tumorigenic segregants. Formal proof of the involvement of the normal chromosome 11 in the suppression of tumorigenicity will depend upon the addition of this chromosome alone to the appropriate hybrid cell lines. The technique of microcell hybridization should provide the methodology for such studies.[69] Saxon et al.[70] have recently shown that individual human chromosomes may be marked with a dominant selective marker and specifically transferred to any human cell.

VI. CONCLUSIONS

The technique of somatic cell hybridization has provided valuable information about the processes by which a normal cell progresses to a malignant one. Studies clearly have shown that tumorigenicity behaves as a recessive genetic trait in mammalian cells. In addition, there appear to be at least two different genes which control the expression of tumorigenicity as evidenced by the ability of two tumorigenic cells to form a non-tumorigenic hybrid cell. This concept is further supported by the evidence of several different human chromosomes which appear to correlate with the ability to suppress tumorigenicity in the hybrid cells. Two more genes also appear to be involved in the control of the transformed phenotype and immortality, respectively.

The data on chromosomes which appear to control the expression of tumorigenicity are consistent with information gathered from other types of studies. Thus Bloch-Shtacher and Sachs[71] have shown that chromosome 3 appeared to be involved in the expression of tumorigenicity in Chinese hamster cells by examining a series of tumorigenic and nontumorigenic sister cell lines. The data from the studies of Klinger and Shows also appear to implicate several of the same human chromosomes as the studies of Stanbridge, Benedict, and their co-workers. These have implicated chromosomes 1, 11, and 13 as potential carriers of recessive cancer genes. These same chromosomes have been associated with several pediatric human cancers, where deletions are often observed in hereditary cases. However, it is interesting to note that homozygosity at the altered locus appears to be necessary for the process of malignant transformation to proceed.[72] The data from human cell hybrid studies have demonstrated that a gene dosage effect occurs in the control of the expression of tumorigenicity. Therefore, a complete loss of normal genetic information is not necessary for re-expression of tumorigenicity to occur in the hybrids. These differences may indicate that there are different genes on the same chromosome involved in the etiology of human cancer.

The next important step is the isolation and characterization of these recessive cancer genes. The function of these genes is still not known, nor have any of their gene products been identified. A clue to their function has been reported recently by Stanbridge and his co-workers.[73] They have shown that hybrid cells between tumorigenic HeLa cells and different normal human cells appear to differentiate upon injection into animals into cells that are similar to the normal parent. Thus, these recessive cancer genes may restore to the tumor cells an ability to respond to a normal differentiation signal in the animal. Comings[74] proposed that cancer may be a loss of expression of regulatory genes whose normal role in cells is in the control of development. The results from the studies on the control of tumorigenicity in somatic cell hybrids provide strong evidence for such a theory. They also emphasize the long-standing relationship between differentiation, cell growth, and malignancy.

REFERENCES

1. Barski, G., Sorieul, S., and Cornefurt, Fr., Production dans des cultures *in vitro* de deux souches cellulaires en association de cellules de caractere "hybride", *C.R. Acad. Sci.,* 251, 1825, 1960.
2. Szybalski, W. S., Szybalska, E. H., and Ragni, G., Genetic studies with human cell lines, *Natl. Cancer Inst. Monogr.,* 7, 75, 1962.
3. Harris, H. and Watkins, J. F., Hybrid cells derived from mouse and man: artificial heterokaryons of mammalian cells from different species, *Nature (London),* 205, 640, 1965.
4. Pontecorvo, G., Production of mammalian somatic cell hybrids by means of polyethylene glycol treatment, *Somat. Cell Genet.,* 1, 397, 1975.
5. Baker, R. M., Brunette, D. M., Mankovitz, R., Thompson, L. A., Whitmore, G. F., Siminovitch, L., and Till, J. E., Ouabain-resistant mutants of mouse and hamster cells in culture, *Cell,* 1, 9, 1974.
6. Harris, H., Some thoughts about genetics, differentiation, and malignancy, *Somat. Cell Genet.,* 6, 923, 1979.
7. Barski, G. and Belehradek, J., Jr., Inheritance of malignancy in somatic cell hybrids, *Somat. Cell Genet.,* 6, 897, 1979.
8. Barski, G., Sorieul, S., and Cornefurt, Fr., "Hybrid" type cells in combined cultures of two different mammalian cell strains, *J. Natl. Cancer Inst.,* 26, 1269, 1961.
9. Barski, G. and Cornefurt, Fr., Characteristics of "hybrid"-type clonal cell lines obtained from mixed cultures *in vitro, J. Natl. Cancer Inst.,* 28, 801, 1962.
10. Harris, H., Miller, O. J., Klein, G., Worst, P., and Tachibana, T., Suppression of malignancy by cell fusion, *Nature (London),* 223, 363, 1969.
11. Klein, G., Bregula, U., Wiener, F., and Harris, H., The analysis of malignancy by cell fusion. I. Hybrids between tumour cells and L cell derivatives, *J. Cell Sci.,* 8, 659, 1971.
12. Berebbi, M. and Barski, G., Hybridation entre deux lignees cellulaires de hamster Chinois a pouvoir tumorigene different, *C.R. Acad. Sci.,* 272, 351, 1971.
13. Sager, R. and Kovac, P. E., Genetic analysis of tumorigenesis. I. Expression of tumor-forming ability in hamster hybrid cell lines, *Somat. Cell Genet.,* 4, 375, 1978.
14. Stanbridge, E. J., Suppression of malignancy in human cells, *Nature (London),* 260, 17, 1976.
15. Croce, C. M., Barrick, J., Linnenbach, A., and Koprowski, H., Expression of malignancy in hybrids between normal and malignant cells, *J. Cell. Physiol.,* 99, 279, 1979.
16. Kucherlapati, R. and Shin, S., Genetic control of tumorigenicity in interspecific mammalian cell hybrids, *Cell,* 16, 639, 1979.
17. Jonasson, J. and Harris, H., The analysis of malignancy by cell fusion. VIII. Evidence for the intervention of an extra-chromosomal element, *J. Cell Sci.,* 24, 255, 1977.
18. Evans, E. P., Burtenshaw, M. D., Brown, B. B., Hennion, R., and Harris, H., The analysis of malignancy by cell fusion. IX. Re-examination and clarification of the cytogenetic problem, *J. Cell Sci.,* 56, 113, 1982.
19. Giacomoni, D., Tumorigenicity and intracisternal A-particle expression of hybrids between murine myeloma and lymphocytes, *Cancer Res.,* 39, 4481, 1979.
20. Weissman, B. E. and Stanbridge, E. J., Complementation of the tumorigenic phenotype in human cell hybrids, *J. Natl. Cancer Inst.,* 70, 667, 1983.
21. Miller, R. A. and Ruddle, F. H., Pluripotent teratocarcinoma-thymus somatic cell hybrids, *Cell,* 9, 45, 1976.
22. Gee, C. J. and Harris, H., Tumorigenicity of cells transformed by simian virus 40 and of hybrids between such cells and normal diploid cells, *J. Cell Sci.,* 36, 223, 1979.
23. Howell, N. and Sager, R., Noncoordinate expression of SV40-induced transformation and tumorigenicity in mouse cell hybrids, *Somat. Cell Genet.,* 5, 129, 1979.
24. Koprowski, H. and Croce, C. M., Tumorigenecity of simian virus 40-transformed human cells and mouse-human hybrids in nude mice, *Proc. Natl. Acad. Sci. U.S.A.,* 74, 1142, 1977.
25. Weissman, B. E. and Stanbridge, E. J., Complexity of control of tumorigenic expression in intraspecies hybrids of human SV40-transformed fibroblasts and normal human fibroblast cell lines, *Cytogenet. Cell Genet.,* 35, 263, 1983.
26. Craig, R. W. and Sager, R., Suppression of tumorigenicity in hybrids of normal and oncogene-transformed CHEF cells, *Proc. Natl. Acad. Sci. U.S.A.,* 82, 2062, 1985.
27. Wiener, F., Klein, G., and Harris, H., The analysis of malignancy by cell fusion. VI. Hybrids between different tumour cells, *J. Cell Sci.,* 16, 189, 1974.
28. Marshall, C. J. and Dave, H., Suppression of the transformed phenotype in somatic cell hybrids, *J. Cell Sci.,* 33, 171, 1978.
29. Geurts van Kessel, A. H. M. G., De Both, N. J., and Hagemeijer, A., Decreased tumorigenicity of Chinese hamster cells after fusion with tumorigenic mouse myeloid leukemia cells, *Cytogenet. Cell Genet.,* 34, 253, 1982.

30. Choi, K.-H., Tevethia, S. S., and Shin, S., Tumor formation by SV40-transformed human cells in nude mice: the role of SV40 T antigens, *Cytogenet. Cell Genet.*, 36, 633, 1983.

31. Straus, D. S., Jonasson, J., and Harris, H., Growth in vitro of tumour cell X fibroblast hybrids in which malignancy is suppressed, *J. Cell Sci.*, 25, 73, 1976.

32. Smith, B. L. and Sager, R., Genetic analysis of tumorigenesis. XXI. Suppressor genes in CHEF cells, *Somat. Cell Mol. Genet.*, 11, 25, 1985.

33. Marshall, C. J., Expression of the transformed phenotype and tumorigenicity in somatic cell hybrids, *J. Cell Sci.*, 39, 319, 1979.

34. Carney, D. N., Edgell, C. J., Gazdar, A. F., and Minna, J. D., Suppression of malignancy in human lung cancer (A549/8) X mouse fibroblast (3T3-4E) somatic cell hybrids, *J. Natl. Cancer Inst.*, 62, 411, 1979.

35. Bramwell, M. E. and Harris, H., An abnormal membrane glycoprotein associated with malignancy in a wide range of tumours, *Proc. R. Soc. London B, Ser.*, 201, 87, 1978.

36. White, M. K., Bramwell, M. E., and Harris, H., Hexose transport in hybrids between malignant and normal cells, *Nature (London)*, 294, 232, 1981.

37. White, M. K., Bramwell, M. E., and Harris, H., Kinetic parameters of hexose transport in hybrids between malignant and non-malignant cells, *J. Cell Sci.*, 62, 49, 1983.

38. Stanbridge, E. J. and Wilkinson, J., Analysis of malignancy in human cells: malignant and transformed phenotypes are under separate genetic control, *Proc. Natl. Acad. Sci. U.S.A.*, 75, 1466, 1978.

39. Klinger, H. P., Suppression of tumorigenicity in somatic cell hybrids. I. Suppression and reexpression of tumorigenicity in diploid human X D98AH2 hybrids and independent segregation of tumorigenicity from other cell phenotypes, *Cytogenet. Cell Genet.*, 27, 254, 1980.

40. Larizza, L., Tenchini, M. L., Mottura, A., De Carli, L., Colombi, M., and Barlati, S., Expression of transformation markers and suppression of tumorigenicity in human cell hybrids, *Eur. J. Cancer Clin. Oncol.*, 18, 845, 1982.

41. Stanbridge, E. J., Der, C. J., Doersen, C. J., Nishimi, R. Y., Peehl, D. M., Weissman, B. E., and Wilkinson, J., Human cell hybrids: analysis of transformation and tumorigenicity, *Science*, 215, 252, 1982.

42. Tenchini, M. L., Larrizza, L., Mottura, A., Colombi, M., Barlati, S., and De Carli, L., Studies on transformation markers and tumorigenicity in segregant clones from a human hybrid line, *Eur. J. Cancer Clin. Oncol.*, 19, 1143, 1983.

43. Der, C. J. and Stanbridge, E. J., A tumour-specific membrane phosphoprotein marker in human cell hybrids, *Cell*, 15, 1241, 1981.

44. Bunn, C. L. and Tarrant, G. M., Limited lifespan in somatic cell hybrids and cybrids, *Exp. Cell Res.*, 127, 385, 1980.

45. Pereira-Smith, O. M. and Smith, J. R., Evidence for the recessive nature of cellular immortality, *Science*, 221, 964, 1983.

46. Silinskas, K. C., Kateley, S. A., Tower, J. E., Maher, V. M., and McCormick, J. J., Induction of anchorage-independent growth in human fibroblasts by propane sulfate, *Cancer Res.*, 41, 1620, 1981.

47. Der, C. J., Krontiris, T. G., and Cooper, G. M., Transforming genes for human bladder and lung carcinoma cell lines are homologous to the *ras* genes of Harvey and Kirsten sarcoma viruses, *Proc. Natl. Acad. Sci. U.S.A.*, 79, 3637, 1982.

48. Goldfarb, M. P., Shimizu, K., Perucho, M., and Wigler, M. H., Isolation and preliminary characterization of a human transforming gene for T24 bladder carcinoma cells, *Nature (London)*, 296, 404, 1982.

49. Pulciani, S., Santos, E., Lauver, A. V., Long, L. K., Robbins, K. C., and Barbacid, M., Oncogenes in human tumor cell lines; molecular cloning of a transforming gene from a human bladder carcinoma cells, *Proc. Natl. Acad. Sci. U.S.A.*, 79, 2845, 1982.

50. Shih, C. and Weinberg, R. A., Isolation of transforming sequence from a human bladder carcinoma cell line, *Cell*, 29, 161, 1982.

51. Gourbin, G., Goldman, D. S., Luce, J., Heiman, P. E., and Cooper, G. M., Molecular cloning and nucleotide sequence of a transforming gene detected by transfection of chicken B-cell lymphoma DNA, *Nature (London)*, 302, 114, 1983.

52. Schechter, A. L., Stern, D. F., Vaidyanathan, L., Decker, S. J., Drebin, J. A., Greene, M. I., and Weinberg, R. A., The *neu* oncogene: an *erb*-B-related gene encoding a 185,000 M_1 tumour antigen, *Nature (London)*, 312, 513, 1984.

53. Lee, W.-H., Murphree, A. L., and Benedict, W. F., Expression and amplification of the N-*myc* gene in primary retinoblastoma, *Nature (London)*, 309, 458, 1984.

54. Pelicci, P.-G., Lanfrancone, L., Brathwaite, M. D., Wolman, S. R., and Dalla-Favera, R., Amplification of the c-*myb* oncogene in a case of human acute myelogenous leukemia, *Science*, 224, 1117, 1984.

55. Little, C. D., Nau, M. M., Carney, D. N., Gazdar, A. F., and Minna, J. D., Amplification and expression of the c-*myc* oncogene in human cancer cell lines, *Nature (London)*, 306, 194, 1983.
56. Marshall, C. J., Hall, A., and Weiss, R. A., A transforming gene present in human sarcoma cell lines, *Nature (London)*, 299, 171, 1982.
57. Benedict, W. F., Weissman, B. E., Mark, C., and Stanbridge, E. J., Tumorigenicity in nude mice of hybrids between the human fibrosarcoma cell line HT-1080 and normal human fibroblasts is gene dose dependent, *Cancer Res.*, 44, 3471, 1984.
58. Weissman, B., Mark, C. F., Benedict, W. F., and Stanbridge, E. J., Expression of the N-ras oncogene in tumorigenic and non-tumorigenic HT 1080 fibrosarcoma X normal human fibroblast hybrid cells, in *Progress in Clinical and Biological Research*, Vol. 175, Evans, A. E., D'Angio, G. J., and Seeger, R. C., Eds., Alan R. Liss, New York, 1985, 141.
59. Geiser, A. G., Der, C. J., Marshall, C. J., and Stanbridge, E. J., Suppression of tumorigenicity with continued expression of the c-Ha-*ras* oncogene in EJ bladder carcinoma x human fibroblast hybrid cells, *Proc. Natl. Acad. Sci. U.S.A.*, 83, 5209, 1986.
60. Charnay, P., Treisman, R., Mellon, P., Chao, M., Axel, R., and Maniatis, T., Differences in human- and -globin gene expression in mouse erythroleukemia cells: the role of intragenic sequences, *Cell*, 38, 251, 1984.
61. Davidson, R. L., Control of expression of differentiated functions in somatic cell hybrids, in *Somatic Cell Hybridisation*, Davidson, R. L. and De la Cruz, F., Eds., Raven Press, New York, 1974, 131.
62. Land, H., Parada, L. F., and Weinberg, R. A., Tumorigenic conversion of primary embryo fibroblasts requires at least two cooperating oncogenes, *Nature (London)*, 304, 596, 1983.
63. Jonasson, J., Povey, S., and Harris, H., The analysis of malignancy by cell fusion. VII. Cytogenetic analysis of hybrids between malignant and diploid cells and of tumours derived from them, *J. Cell Sci.*, 24, 217, 1977.
64. Marshall, C. J., Expression of the transformed phenotype and tumorigenicity in somatic cell hybrids, *J. Cell Sci.*, 39, 319, 1979.
65. Harrison, J. J., Anisowicz, A., Gadi, I. K., Raffeld, M., and Sager, R., Azacytidine-induced tumorigenesis of CHEF/18 cells: correlated DNA methylation and chromosome changes, *Proc. Natl. Acad. Sci. U.S.A.*, 80, 6606, 1983.
66. Klinger, H. P. and Shows, T. B., Suppression of tumorigenicity in somatic cell hybrids. II. Human chromosomes implicated as suppressors of tumorigenicity in hybrids with Chinese hamster ovary cells, *J. Natl. Cancer Inst.*, 71, 559, 1983.
67. Stanbridge, E. J., Flandermeyer, R. R., Daniels, D. W., and Nelson-Rees, W. A., Specific chromosome loss associated with the expression of tumorigenicity in human cell hybrids, *Somat. Cell Genet.*, 7, 699, 1981.
68. Srivatsan, E. S., Krontiris, T. G., Benedict, W. F., and Stanbridge, E. J., Molecular analysis of the chromosomal control of neoplastic expression in human cell hybrids: chromosome 11 is implicated in the suppression of tumorigenicity, *Cancer Res.*, in press.
69. Fournier, R. E. K. and Ruddle, F. H., Microcell-mediated transfer of murine chromosomes into mouse, Chinese hamster and human somatic cells, *Proc. Natl. Acad. Sci. U.S.A.*, 74, 319, 1977.
70. Saxon, P. J., Srivatsan, E. S., Leipzig, G. V., Sameshima, J. H., and Stanbridge, E. J., Selective transfer of individual human chromosomes to recipient cells, *Mol. Cell. Biol.*, 5, 140, 1985.
71. Bloch-Shtacher, N. and Sachs, L., Identification of a chromosome that controls malignancy in Chinese hamster cells, *J. Cell. Physiol.*, 93, 205, 1977.
72. Murphree, A. L. and Benedict, W. F., Retinoblastoma: clues to human oncogenesis, *Science*, 223, 1028, 1984.
73. Stanbridge, E. J., Fagg, B. A., and Der, C. J., Differentiation and the control of tumorigenicity in human cell hybrids, in *Human Carcinogenesis*, Harris, C. and Autrup, H., Eds., Academic Press, New York, 1983, 97.
74. Comings, D. E., A general theory of carcinogenesis, *Proc. Natl. Acad. Sci. U.S.A.*, 70, 3324, 1973.
75. Scaletta, L. J. and Ephrussi, B., Hybridization of normal and neoplastic cells in vitro, *Nature (London)*, 205, 1169, 1965.
76. Defendi, V., Ephrussi, B., Koprowski, H., and Yoshida, M. C., Properties of hybrids between polyoma-transformed and normal mouse cell lines, *Proc. Natl. Acad. Sci. U.S.A.*, 57, 299, 1967.
77. Silagi, S., Hybridization of a malignant melanoma cell line with L cells in vitro, *Cancer Res.*, 27, 1953, 1967.
78. Ruddle, F. H., Chen, T., Shows, T. B., and Silagi, S., Interstrain somatic cell hybrids in the mouse, *Exp. Cell. Res.*, 60, 139, 1970.
79. Aden, D. P. and Knowles, B. P., Tumorigenicity of intraspecific somatic cell hybrids in nude mice, *J. Natl. Cancer Inst.*, 58, 743, 1977.
80. Aviles, D., Jami, J., Rousset, J., and Ritz, E., Tumor x host cell hybrids in the mouse: chromosomes from the normal parent maintained in malignant hybrid tumors, *J. Natl. Cancer Inst.*, 58, 1391, 1977.

81. Halaban, R., Nordlund, J., Francke, U., Moellman, G., and Eisenstadt, J. M., Supermelanotic hybrids derived from mouse melanomas and normal mouse cells, *Somat. Cell Genet.,* 6, 29, 1980.
82. Bregula, U., Klein, G., and Harris, H., The analysis of malignancy by cell fusion. II. Hybrids between Ehrlich cells and normal diploid cells, *J. Cell Sci.,* 8, 673, 1971.
83. Wiener, F., Klein, G., and Harris, H., The analysis of malignancy by cell fusion. III. Hybrids between diploid fibroblasts and other tumour cells, *J. Cell Sci.,* 8, 681, 1971.
84. Kao, F. and Hartz, J. A., Genetic and tumorigenic characteristics of cell hybrids formed between injected tumor cells and host cells, *J. Natl. Cancer Inst.,* 59, 409, 1977.
85. Peehl, D. M. and Stanbridge, E. J., The role of differentiation in the control of tumorigenic expression in human cell hybrids, *Int. J. Cancer,* 30, 113, 1982.
86. Weissman, B. E., unpublished data, 1985.
87. Stanbridge, E. J., personal communication, 1985.
88. Barski, G., Blanchard, M.-G., Youn, J. K., and Leon, B., Expression of malignancy in interspecies Chinese hamster x mouse cell hybrids, *J. Natl. Cancer Inst.,* 51, 781, 1973.
89. Schafer, R., Doehmer, J., Druge, P. M., Rademacher, I., and Willecke, K., Genetic analysis of transformed and malignant phenotypes in somatic cell hybrids between tumorigenic Chinese hamster cells and diploid mouse cell fibroblasts, *Cancer Res.,* 41, 1214, 1981.
90. Bordelon, M. R., Shows, T. B., Chen, T. R., and Stubblefield, E., Correlation of in vivo malignancy with in vitro properties of human-mouse hybrid cells, *J. Natl. Cancer Inst.,* 56, 499, 1976.
91. Rose, C. J. and Rose, G. B., Suppression of malignancy in mouse-man hybrid cells, *Pathology,* 10, 343, 1978.
92. Klinger, H. P., Baim, A. S., Eun, C. K., Shows, T. B., and Ruddle, F. H., Human chromosomes which affect tumorigenicity in hybrids of diploid human with heteroploid human or rodent cells, *Cytogenet. Cell Genet.,* 22, 245, 1978.
93. Geurts van Kessel, A. H. M., den Boer, W. C., van Agthoven, A. J., and Hagemeijer, A., Decreased tumorigenicity of rodent cells after fusion with leukocytes from normal and leukemic donors, *Somat. Cell Genet.,* 7, 645, 1981.

Chapter 4

THE REGULATION OF GENE EXPRESSION BY TUMOR PROMOTERS

Timothy H. Carter

TABLE OF CONTENTS

I. INTRODUCTION

The aims of this chapter are to review the evidence for modulation of gene expression by tumor promoters, and to describe our present understanding of the mechanism by which promoting agents cause these changes. The focus will be on primary effects of tumor promoters — changes in gene expression that occur within hours, or in some cases minutes, after exposure to these agents. Later changes in gene expression, which may be crucial to the phenomena of transformation, promotion, or progression, are likely to be pleiotropic responses to the altered phenotype of the "promoted" cell. Given our present lack of knowledge about the pathways of gene expression during promotion, these secondary responses are thus less easily accessible to biochemical analysis than are the initial effects which occur in a cell that has not yet been exposed experimentally to a promoting agent.

It should be noted at the outset that a potential problem with attempting to understand the action of tumor promoters by isolating their primary epigenetic effects is that by definition the phenomenon of promotion, even in vitro, occurs in a population of cells that has been severely stressed. Exposure to carcinogens, whether physical, chemical, or biological (e.g., viruses) results in profound, short-term changes in cellular physiology, which are followed by genetic alterations that may cause equally severe, lasting changes. In the case of physical and chemical carcinogens particularly, initial cellular changes are nonlocalized and often unpredictable. From this standpoint, cells infected by oncogenic viruses may afford the best opportunity to observe the action of tumor promoters in a controlled way that is also relevant to oncogenesis, because these biological carcinogens operate according to a reproducible genetic program which is itself accessible to detailed analysis and experimental manipulation. Nevertheless, progress in understanding the primary effects of tumor promoters on gene expression has been made during the past several years in a variety of systems, including fibroblast cell cycle control, tumor cell differentiation, and viral gene expression in both chronically and acutely infected cells. Much of the data document a rapid effect by tumor-promoting agents on transcription of a limited set of genes related to cell growth and differentiation, or to early stages of viral replication. Modulation of the expression of cellular genes by tumor promoters presumably leads to survival and proliferation of initiated cells, thereby allowing time for secondary genetic changes to occur which fix the altered growth phenotype.

II. EVIDENCE FOR MODULATION OF CELLULAR GENE EXPRESSION

A. In Vivo Studies

In the decades since its development, the "two-stage" mouse-skin carcinogenesis assay,[1,2] described in detail elsewhere in these volumes, has become the "classical" paradigm for the study of tumor promotion. In this assay, mouse skin is exposed to an initiating carcinogen, usually in a single dose, followed by repeated applications of a second agent. The second agent is defined as a promoter if it is not carcinogenic when applied alone, and either (1) it causes the accelerated appearance of tumors, or the appearance of tumors in a higher proportion of animals than would otherwise be expected from the initiating carcinogen (in this case, a "complete" carcinogen); or (2) it causes tumors in the case where the initiating carcinogen alone is unable to do so (i.e., an "incomplete" carcinogen).

Application of tumor promoters to mouse epidermis causes rapid changes in macromolecular synthesis that are indicative of increased gene expression. Experiments to define global effects showed that both RNA[3,178] and protein synthesis[4] were stimulated. In an interesting, and so far unique, study to examine macromolecular synthesis in precancerous (as opposed to normal) mouse skin that was subsequently exposed to a tumor promoter, mice were injected subcutaneously with 3-methylcholanthrene and exposed to 12-O-tetradecanoyl-phorbol-13-acetate (TPA) for from 3 to 96 hr.[5] Macromolecular synthesis in epidermis, dermis, and subcutis was measured by incorporation of radiolabeled precursors. Overall RNA synthesis in initiated tissues remained relatively unchanged, but several waves of DNA synthesis and cell division were detected, as well as the appearance of new protein. Promoted tissues, however, were stimulated early to synthesize all three classes of macromolecules; DNA synthesis in these cells was markedly altered in temporal pattern and intensity, compared to initiated cells that were not exposed to a promoter. The authors concluded that TPA recruited preneoplastic cells to DNA synthesis, thereby accelerating their proliferation. Because it is now possible to detect small amounts of gene products that are associated with tumor-promoter action (e.g., cellular proto-oncogenes — see Section II.C), use of initiated in vivo systems to study the modulation of expression of such genes could provide further insight into the phenomenon of tumor promotion, as distinct from the biochemical effects of tumor promoters.

The first attempts to relate the synthesis of specific polypeptides to tumor-promoter action identified two polypeptides that were detectable only in extracts of mouse skin exposed to TPA.[6-9] Although promoting agents alone do not cause tumors, some of these agents are mitogenic, causing localized hyperplasia, and all seem to be irritants.[4,10-14] Comparative in vivo studies of gene activity modulated in response to tumor promoters must therefore control the biologic effects of these agents that might not be relevant to tumor promotion. In a recent study to identify changes in the synthesis of epidermal proteins in response to promoters, two-dimensional polyacrylamide gel electrophoresis of polypeptides labeled with ^{35}S-methionine in mice exposed locally to TPA or the second-stage promoter, mezerein, showed neosynthesis of several polypeptides as early as 3 hr after exposure to the promoter.[15] These changes were a specific response to the promoter in that they were different from those induced by agents causing hyperplasia, but inactive as tumor promoters (acetic acid, ethylphenylpropionate, turpentine, and the calcium ionophore A23187). The changes also were prevented by fluocinolone acetonide, an agent that interferes with tumor promotion.[16] Of 11 polypeptides that showed obvious TPA-specific changes in incorporation of radioactivity during a 4-hr labeling period, 8 were thought to be related to keratin by comparison of electrophoretic mobilities. Labeling of four of these keratin-like polypeptides, all with similar molecular weight but differing in charge, decreased by a factor of ten or more. Of the remaining four keratin-like polypeptides, three (51, 56, and 54 kdaltons) were labeled only in TPA-treated cells, and a fourth increased by a factor of five at 3 hr after exposure to TPA. These effects on keratin-like polypeptides are probably related to the ability of phorbol ester tumor promoters to facilitate the differentiative pathway in a subpopulation of epithelial cells.[17] Of the two nonkeratin polypeptides labeled more strongly in promoted epidermis than in controls, one acidic polypeptide (12 kdalton) was increased by a factor of five at 3 hr, and a new basic polypeptide (41 kdalton) appeared by 24 hr (see Table 1). One 52 kdalton basic polypeptide decreased 20-fold by 3 hr after promotion. The mechanisms underlying the changes in labeling of these polypeptides were not addressed in this study. Such changes could have resulted from differences either in rates of synthesis or in stability.

Although it has not yet been determined how many of the TPA-induced polypeptides in mouse skin are products of transcriptional or posttranscriptional regulation, it is likely that at least some of them are products of neotranscription. Sauer[182] and his

Table 1

INDUCTION OF POLYPEPTIDE SYNTHESIS IN MOUSE CELLS BY
TUMOR PROMOTERS

Gene product	Time of appearance[a]	System	Ref.
Keratin-like polypeptides	3—24 hr	Epidermis	6—9, 15, 70
12 kdalton, acidic	3 hr	Epidermis	15
41 kdalton, basic	24 hr	Epidermis	15
32 kdalton, gp (cytoskeletal or membrane-associated)	2 hr	Balb/c 3T3	39, 65
35 kdalton, gp (MEP)	6 hr	MEF	41, 66, 67, 70
25 kdalton, unstable	6 hr	MEF	70
50 kdalton, unstable	1 hr	MEF	70
β actin	5 min	Balb/c 3T3	96
c-fos	5 min	Balb/c 3T3	96-99
c-myc	2 hr	Balb/c 3T3	96, 97
Ornithine decarboxylase, S-adenosyl methionine decarboxylase		Epidermis	13, 18, 27—29
		Skin cells	18, 27
Histidine decarboxylase		Epidermis	21, 22
cAMP-phosphodiesterase		Epidermis	23, 24
Ribosomal proteins		Epidermis	25
Histones		Epidermis	26, 27
Epidermal transglutaminase		Basal skin cells	17, 29, 40, 71—75

Note: MEF, mouse embryo fibroblasts.

[a]   Where no time is given, increases were observed within 12 hr after exposure to a promoter.

colleagues have recently identified more than 50 cDNA clones from among reverse transcripts of the total polyadenylated RNA population in mouse carcinomas induced by dimethylbenzanthracine (DMBA) and TPA that represent RNA species with altered abundances in the tumor cells. When two of these clones corresponding to genetic sequences expressed in high abundance in carcinomas were used to screen Northern blots of mRNA from mouse skin that had been exposed to TPA, both clones detected RNA that was newly transcribed within 2 hr after TPA treatment. The sizes of the RNA molecules, 1.1 and 2.7 kilobases (kb), are in principle large enough to encode any of the mouse epidermal polypeptides whose synthesis was reported to be increased in response to promoters.[15]

A number of enzyme activities and identifiable nonenzymatic proteins has been found to increase in mouse skin, as well as in cells from other species after exposure to promoting agents: ornithine decarboxylase (ODC) and S-adenosyl-methionine decarboxylase,[18] phospholipase A2,[19,20] histidine decarboxylase,[21,22] cyclic AMP-phosphodiesterase,[23,24] ribosomal proteins,[25] and histones.[7,26]

ODC has received the majority of attention over the past decade because it was the first to be discovered,[18] is readily assayed, and is associated with biochemical events leading to DNA replication and cell proliferation.[27] In mouse skin, ODC activity was induced by TPA[18,27,28] and aplysiatoxin, a polyacetate tumor promoter;[13] induction was enhanced by corticosteroids,[29] and is rapid and transient. In rat skin, increased enzyme activity was apparent by 3 hr, reached a peak at 4 hr, and fell to control levels by 12 hr.[30] After i.p. administration of TPA or phenobarbital (a weak promoter) to rats, liver ODC increased with similar kinetics.[31] The increase in ODC activity was prevented by pretreatment with actinomycin D[30,31] or cycloheximide,[30] implicating induction at the level of transcription rather than activation of pre-existing enzyme or translation of cryptic mRNA.

Relatively little work has been done on the other enzymes. Histidine decarboxylase activity was induced in mouse skin by indole alkaloid promoters[21] and TPA.[22] In the latter case, it appeared that the target cell in the dermis was a nonbasophilic lymphocyte of bone marrow origin. Cyclic AMP-phosphodiesterase activity was found to increase modestly 13 hr after phorbol ester treatment, and the magnitude of the increase paralleled the tumor-promoting activity of the doses and compounds employed. Interestingly, the induction of this enzyme was prevented by colchicine and vinblastine, drugs which interfere with microtubule function. In light of observations that cytoskeletal alterations are among the first cytologically apparent consequences of tumor-promoter action,[32,33] it is possible that these structural elements are not only targets, but also mediators of the effect of tumor promoters on gene expression. Carter et al.[34,35] have found that disruption of microtubules also prevents acceleration of the human adenovirus genetic program by TPA in HeLa cells (see Section III.B.3.b).

B. In Vitro Studies
1. Tumor-Promoter Effects on Untransformed Cell Lines

The ability to study the complex interactions between target cells and tumor promoters has been aided by the identification or development of well-defined cell culture systems responsive to these agents.[17,36-43] These systems fall into four categories: (1) in vitro analogs of two-step carcinogenesis;[36] (2) "normal", untransformed cells in which the response to tumor promoters alone is studied;[17] (3) virally or chemically transformed cells in which expression of viral or cellular oncogenes is monitored after exposure to a promoting agent;[44] and (4) tumor cells from specific tissues that can be induced to differentiate or de-differentiate by tumor promoters.[45]

Two-stage carcinogenesis studies in cell culture have shown that tumor promoters can enhance transformation induced by a variety of chemical and physical agents.[36,37,44] For example, TPA promotes transformation by chemical carcinogens,[46,47] UV light,[48] and X-irradiation.[49] In addition, TPA has been shown to increase the frequency of cell transformation by a number of viruses, among them human type-5 adenovirus,[44,50,51] SV40,[52,53] polyoma,[54] Epstein-Barr virus,[55] and bovine papilloma virus.[56] Thus, cell culture systems would seem to provide reasonable in vitro analogs to the in vivo action of promoting agents.

The first attempts to identify gene products induced by tumor promoters in cell culture documented the induction of ODC, which was also the first biochemical activity to be identified as an early target of modulation in mouse skin.[18,27] Studies on primary and transformed hamster cells showed a dose-dependent stimulation of enzyme activity that attained a maximum between 4 and 6 hr after exposure to TPA, and a synergistic effect of serum factors.[57] Transformed hamster cells were more responsive to stimulation than were primary cells.[57,58] Interestingly, a similar observation was made for cells of human origin: ODC was readily induced in HeLa cells by phorbol-12,13-dibutyrate,[59] but not by TPA in human skin fibroblasts.[28] Induction of ODC in response to tumor promoters is clearly dependent on species, as well as cell type. Activity was stimulated in Balb c/3T3[28] and Reuber H35 hepatoma[60] lines, but not in rat embryo fibroblasts.[28]

The biochemical mechanism of ODC induction in cell culture has not been elucidated. Retinoids were found to block induction,[61] corroborating the observation in mouse skin, but the mechanistic significance of this consistent antagonism of retinoids is unclear. Use of several Chinese hamster ovary cell mutants with altered cyclic AMP-dependent protein kinase activity indicated that induction of ODC by TPA was partially inhibited in these cells, but was less sensitive than induction of ODC by cholera toxin.[42] The results were taken to suggest that cAMP-dependent kinase activity was not essential to induction of ODC by phorbol ester tumor promoters. However, the data are equally consistent with the possibility that cAMP-dependent kinase activity is one of several components that can mediate the TPA effect.

Given that both actinomycin D and cycloheximide block induction of ODC by tumor promoters in vivo,[30,31] it is reasonable to conclude that induction of this enzyme results from increased transcription of the ODC gene within the first few hours after treatment. This recently has been confirmed by direct measurement of the ODC transcription rate in PC12 cells exposed to TPA.[181] Recent purification of the ODC protein[177] should allow functional measurement of ODC mRNA levels by cell-free translation and immunological detection. The significance of ODC stimulation by tumor promoters has been assumed to be that the induction of the enzyme is involved in steps leading to DNA replication, and therefore to cell proliferation. Although this may be true in many cases, at least one set of data suggests that this connection may not be obligatory. O'Brien et al.[28] reported that TPA induced DNA synthesis in human fibroblasts without affecting ODC levels. However, given the dependence of biochemical responses to tumor promoters on cell type and culture conditions (for example, the difference between serum-starved and exponentially growing fibroblasts — see below), the importance of ODC activity in the cellular response to tumor promoters remains a possibility.

Studies of gene expression in mouse cell lines have led to the identification of a number of other gene products whose synthesis is both increased and decreased in response to tumor promoters. Dion et al.[62,63] found that TPA inhibited the synthesis of collagen in JB-6 cells as early as 6 hr after treatment. The decrease in collagen synthesis could be explained by inhibition at a pretranslational stage, because a reduced amount of procollagen mRNA was detected by hybridization and cell-free translation 24 hr after treatment with TPA.[64] In Balb/c 3T3 cells, Hiwasa and colleagues[65] have characterized a 32 kdalton polypeptide whose rate of synthesis is doubled 2 hr after exposure to tumor-promoting phorbol esters, indole alkaloids, or polyacetates; the same polypeptide is unaffected by nonpromoting phorbol esters. This polypeptide was immunologically distinguishable[39] from another TPA-stimulated polypeptide of similar size ("MEP") in mouse epidermal cells described previously by Gottesman.[41,66,67] The partition of the Balb/c 32 kdalton peptide into detergent extracts, and its presence in the particulate fraction of isotonically disrupted cells,[39] suggested that it was associated with the cytoskeleton or membrane, and the fact that it could not be enzymatically iodinated in intact cells indicated that it was not exposed on the cell surface. The increased synthesis of this polypeptide after TPA treatment was prevented by actinomycin D, coupled with the increased amount of translatable mRNA for the 32-kdalton product found after TPA treatment; it is thus likely that the gene for this polypeptide, like that for MEP, is regulated transcriptionally by TPA.

The development of a mouse epidermal cell culture model,[40] and of techniques for the selective cultivation of basal cells from mouse skin,[68] has led to the identification of additional gene products whose expression is associated with exposure of primary mouse skin cells to tumor promoters. Gottesman[67] has reported the increased synthesis of a small excreted glycoprotein (MEP) in transformed cells. The abundance of messenger RNA for this protein increases within the first 6 hr after TPA treatment of mouse epidermal cells, indicating pretranslational regulation. The purified glycoprotein, with an apparent molecular weight of 35 kdalton, binds to concanavalin A columns, and has an unglycosylated molecular weight of 33 kdalton.[66] Among the surface glycoproteins of 3T3 cells, the secretion of one, with an apparent molecular weight of 45 kdalton, has been found to decrease after TPA treatment.[69]

Table 2
INDUCTION OF GENES BY TUMOR PROMOTERS IN
OTHER SPECIES

Product	Cell line	Ref.
Multiple polypeptides	Chick-embryo fibroblasts	81
Collagenase	Rabbit synovial fibroblasts	38, 78—80
Prolactin	Clonal rat pituitary tumor	105
Plasminogen activator	Human Bowes melanoma	91
	HeLa	89
Calcitonin	Human medullary thyroid carcinoma	92
UV-induced polypeptides	Human fibroblasts	83
c-fos	Human leukemia	113
ODC	HeLa	59
	Rat	30, 31
	Hamster	42, 57, 58
Phospholipase A2	Canine (MDCK)	19
	Chick-embryo fibroblasts	20

Identification of TPA-induced proteins in mouse epidermal cells by two-dimensional polyacrylamide gel analysis of ^{35}S-methionine labeled extracts showed five polypeptides with increased rates of synthesis within 6 hr of exposure to TPA.[70] The increase was transient, since the rates of synthesis returned to normal by 24 hr. All appeared from pulse-chase experiments to be primary products of translation, and comparison of the gel patterns from two strains of mice showed no differences, an observation that was considered to rule out the possibility that some of the proteins were encoded by endogenous retroviruses. Three of the polypeptides were only detected in TPA-treated cells (25, 55, and 70 kdalton), and the two others had substantially increased rates of synthesis after TPA treatment (35 and 50 kdalton). The 25- and 50-kdalton polypeptides turned over rapidly during a chase. The 55-kdalton product was a phosphoprotein, and the 50-kdalton polypeptide was the most rapidly affected by TPA, increasing in rate of synthesis within 1 hr of exposure. The investigators tentatively identified two of the polypeptides as cytoskeleton-related (55 and 70 kdalton), and the 35-kdalton polypeptide had properties consistent with those of the MEP protein.

In a series of studies on the response of mouse epidermal basal cells to tumor promoters, Yuspa and his colleagues[17,29,40,71-75] have begun to dissect the alternative programs of gene expression leading to differentiation or proliferation. Basal cells grown in low-calcium medium can be induced to differentiate by increase the calcium concentration to 1.2 mM, resulting in reduced DNA synthesis, induction of epidermal transglutaminase, and eventual sloughing of keratinized cells. TPA is able to accelerate this differentiative process, but seemingly only in a subpopulation of basal cells that has been committed to this pathway. In other cells, TPA stimulates division and inhibits differentiation. Induction of ornithine decarboxylase by TPA in basal cell cultures presumably occurs in this latter population, although there is no direct evidence of this. TPA also inhibited the appearance of differentiated cell-specific products in chick-embryo myotubes.[76,77]

Normal and transformed cells from species other than the mouse and hamster have also been shown to respond to tumor promoters by altering the synthesis of various gene products (Table 2). Rabbit synovial fibroblasts growing in monolayer can be induced to synthesize collagenase 6 to 12 hr after treatment,[38,78-80] as well as a 51-kdalton metalloprotein and an unidentified 47-kdalton polypeptide.[80] Corticosteroids enhance the induction of collagenase, and retinoids inhibit it.[79] Induction appears to be at the level of transcription, or at least to be pretranslational, because the effect is inhibited by α amanitin, and can be detected by cell-free translation of mRNA isolated after TPA treatment.[38] Avian cells also show a number of changes in labeling and phosphorylation of polypeptides on two-dimensional polyacrylamide gels after exposure to TPA.[81]

The sole exception to the pattern of selective gene activation by tumor promoters occurs in primary human epidermal cells, which do not show typical biochemical responses such as ODC induction, or increased deoxyglucose uptake.[28,82] There is one report, however, suggesting that culture conditions may play a subtle role in determining responsiveness of primary human cells to phorbol esters, although this possibility has not yet been confirmed by biochemical studies. Primary human skin fibroblasts were found to attain significantly higher saturation densities in response to phorbol-12,13-didecanoate only if the medium contained higher concentrations of certain amino acids.[179] TPA and UV light induce the same 8 polypeptides in human fibroblasts within 2 hr of exposure.[83] Interestingly, the irradiated cells secreted a soluble factor, presumably a polypeptide, which also induced the same products. The tumor-promotion inhibitor, fluocinolone acetonide, prevents the response to the factor, TPA, or irradiation.[83] In mouse-human hybrids, transcription of repressed ribosomal genes by RNA polymerase III was also stimulated by TPA.[84]

2. Tumor-Promoter Effects on Transformed Cell Lines

Cell lines derived from murine lymphomas and leukemias respond to tumor promoters by expressing a variety of genes. The EL4 T-cell lymphoma line synthesizes interleukin-2 mRNA after exposure to TPA.[85] In this case, specific mRNA was quantitated by translation of total polyadenylated RNA in *Xenopus laevis* oocytes and by biologic and chromatographic characterization of the products. Mouse myeloid leukemia cells exposed to TPA and analyzed by two-dimensional polypeptide gels and cell-free translation of mRNA show evidence of altered gene expression at both transcriptional and posttranscriptional levels.[86-88] Induction of the differentiative pathway in these cells by macrophage- and granulocyte-inducing protein caused a similar array of changes which differed in pattern from those induced by TPA.

Transformed human cells respond more typically than primary cells to tumor promoters.[59,89-91] Human medullary thyroid carcinoma cell lines secrete calcitonin in inverse relationship to their virulence. TPA and phorbol-12,13-dibutyrate both enhanced calcitonin secretion sevenfold within 15 min, and calcitonin mRNA levels approximately twofold at 6 hr in a highly tumorigenic line, along with altering its morphology so as to more nearly resemble less virulent, more highly "differentiated" cells.[92] In this context, it is interesting that the concentration of *c-myc* RNA decreased 80% in the same cells after TPA treatment, which is consistent with the idea that *c-myc* expression is a characteristic of proliferating, rather than of differentiating, cells.[93,94] A decline in expression of another oncogene, *c-myb*, has also been reported during differentiation of human myeloblastic leukemia cells after treatment with TPA.[95] In contrast, TPA caused a delayed induction of *c-myc* in untransformed 3T3 cells (see Section II.C).[96-99] The human Bowes melanoma cell line can be induced by TPA to secrete increased amounts of plasminogen activator within 3 hr after exposure.[91] This effect probably results from an increased production of mRNA for plasminogen activator, because it can be prevented by actinomycin D and can be detected by cell-free translation of purified mRNA. Plasminogen activator is also induced by TPA in HeLa cells.[89]

Clonal rat pituitary tumor lines are induced to synthesize prolactin mRNA after exposure to TPA in a manner similar to the effect of thyrotropin-releasing hormone and epidermal growth factor (EGF).[100-104] Supowit et al.[105] have recently succeeded in demonstrating that DNA sequences to the 5′ side of the prolactin gene confer the property of inducibility not only by EGF, but also by TPA.[105] They inserted the flanking sequences in front of the rat growth hormone gene (*grl*) on a pSV$_{2neo}$ plasmid, transfected human A431 cells, and showed that both EGF and TPA induced *grl* transcripts, but not *neo* transcripts, in stably transfected lines. Plasmids containing the entire prolactin gene were also induced with the same kinetics (increased transcription was detectable by 6 hr and maximal, showing a 3.5-fold induction, by 16 to 24 hr). On the other hand, the cloned growth hormone gene itself was not inducible in transfectants. This represents compelling evidence that rapid effects of tumor promoters on gene expression include the enhanced transcription of a restricted set of genes, and that the property of inducibility is inherent in the DNA sequence information of the genes themselves. Interestingly, DNA sequence analysis of the 5′ flanking region of the rat prolactin gene has led to the suggestion that this region might have been acquired by an insertional event during evolution.[106] If this were so, it implies a common origin for regulatory sequences that respond to tumor promoters, and provides an additional rationale for a search for these sequences among cloned genes from various sources. One obvious approach would be to use the prolactin flanking sequences to probe genomic libraries. Candidate sequences could then be tested functionally by construction of chimeric genes and either transfection, or, potentially, by testing their ability to serve as a template for transcription in in vitro systems from promoted cells.

The use of transformed cell lines to study the effects of tumor promoters on gene expression raises obvious questions about the relevance of such effects to the phenomenon of tumor promotion. Observations on a cell that has passed beyond the stage of promotion, or may indeed be permanently "promoted", might focus attention on events and pathways unrelated to the main issue. Nevertheless, the convenience of such systems in providing both ample material and a certain amount of biological uniformity makes these systems attractive targets for biochemical analysis. Fortunately, a number of cases have emerged in which gene expression induced by tumor promoters in transformed cells has an analog in their "normal" counterparts. These include the synthesis of surface-associated glycoproteins disucssed earlier, such as MEP, and the activation or modulation of cellular oncogenes.

C. Modulation of Oncogene Expression by Tumor Promoters

In tests of the ability of TPA to activate tyrosine-specific protein kinases encoded by the chick-embryo *c-src* gene or the avian sarcoma virus (ASV) *v-src,* no conclusive evidence was obtained for any effect.[81,107] Although as early as 1 hr after exposure to TPA it was possible to detect a three- to eightfold stimulation of IgG phosphorylation in immunoprecipitates using anti-p60^{src} antisera,[107] TPA did not enhance ASV kinase activity in infected cells. Furthermore, after TPA treatment of chick-embryo fibroblasts, enhanced phosphorylation of the putative cellular target for *src*-associated kinase (a 34- to 36-kdalton protein) was not detected, and the phosphotyrosine content of cellular polypeptides did not increase.[81]

However, one of the cellular oncogenes has turned out to be among the earliest detectable genetic targets of the action of phorbol ester tumor promoters, as well as of polypeptide growth hormones. This gene is known as *c-fos* for its homology with, and presumed evolutionary relationship to, the transforming oncogene *v-fos* carried by FBJ-osteosarcoma virus.[108-111] *C-fos* is normally expressed in extraembryonal tissues, and in neonatal bone and skin.[112] During a search for genes that might be responsible for cell cycle control in 3T3 cells, Greenberg and Ziff,[96] and other investigators,[97,98] independently turned up *c-fos* as the major, immediate target of regulation in response to polypeptide growth hormones, serum, and TPA. When serum-starved 3T3 cells were fed medium containing any of these factors, the rate of *c-fos* transcription increased dramatically in nuclei isolated as early as 15 min after stimulation.[96] The sequences of c-fos were also detected by Northern blot analysis of polyadenylated cytoplasmic RNA prepared at this time from serum-stimulated cells.[96,97] The kinetics of c-fos transcription following serum addition showed a nearly tenfold stimulation as early as 5 min. Peak rates were attained at 10 min, after which transcription rapidly decreased until it was barely detectable 1 hr after serum stimulation;[96] the concentration of c-fos RNA in cytoplasm peaked at 30 min and persisted until 90 min, although it fell to undetectable levels by 2 hr.

Induction of c-fos was not peculiar to 3T3 cells; rapid induction of c-fos protein was also demonstrated by immunofluorescence in mouse-embryo fibroblasts.[97] A second, fos-related transcript has been identified in Balb/c 3T3 cells stimulated by platelet derived growth factor (PDGF),[99] raising the possibility that multiple c-fos-related genes might be induced by TPA in a given cell type. A c-fos proto-oncogene is expressed in human monocytic and monomyelocytic tumor cell lines[113] when either of these lines is induced by TPA to differentiate into macrophages. As in 3T3 cells, human c-fos mRNA appears within 20 min. Unlike 3T3 cells, however, this RNA persists for over 100 hr, although synthesis of the c-fos polypeptide ceases after 2 hr. In contrast to c-fos, RNA from the oncogene c-myb disappeared between 4 and 8 hr after TPA treatment, correlating with cessation of cell division. Induction of the HL-60 myelocytic line by dimethyl sulfoxide (DMSO), which leads to granulocytic differentiation, did not cause increased c-fos expression.[113]

The one other cellular gene among those tested that was found to be affected as rapidly as c-fos was the gene for β-actin,[96] implying a mechanism that involves, at least initially, the same components as the stimulation of c-fos. Induction of β-actin transcription measured by the nuclear runoff assay was transient, and occurred with kinetics similar to those of c-fos after stimulation by both PDGF and TPA. In the case of stimulation by serum, however, the rate of β-actin transcription was elevated for up to 4 hr and returned to unstimulated rates by 8 hr. It is possible that this difference reflects an additional level of either transcriptional or early posttranscriptional regulation.

Transcription of a second oncogene associated with cell growth control, c-myc,[93,94] also increased transiently in 3T3 cells in response to both growth factors and TPA, but its kinetics lagged behind those of c-fos. Transcription of c-myc peaked at 2 hr and returned to normal by 4 hr,[96] and the cytoplasmic RNA for c-myc persisted for at least 12 hr.[97] Most of the changes in c-fos, c-myc, and β-actin transcription preceded the onset of DNA synthesis in stimulated 3T3 cells which occurred between 10 and 12 hr after addition of the growth factors or TPA. It is tempting to speculate that the induction of c-myc by TPA or growth factors is caused by the fos gene product directly, or by some pleiotropic effect of the fos protein. However, superinduction of both c-fos and c-myc in cells treated with cycloheximide[94,97-99,113] or anisomycin[181] makes this pathway unlikely. As noted earlier, the effect of TPA on c-myc expression in transformed cells is often the opposite of that seen in fibroblasts such as 3T3. These observations are consistent with the hypothesis that the induction of cell proliferation by TPA is accompanied by increased expression of c-myc, whereas induction of differentiation, which leads to cessation of cell division, is associated with reduced c-myc expression.

Among a group of genes tested for regulation in response to growth factors, including 17 oncogenes, the transformation-associated cell protein p53, the genes for β actin, and α tubulin, histone H-3, and dihydrofolate reductase, only transcription of c-fos, c-myc, and β actin was unambiguously stimulated in quiescent 3T3 cells by TPA and peptide growth factors.[96] RNA hybridizing to two other cloned oncogenes, c-myb and *c-fgr*, was synthesized preferentially in nuclei from stimulated cells, but additional cell sequences contained in the cloned probes make interpretation of these data difficult.[96] Oncogenes unequivocally *not* affected by serum (and therefore, presumably not by TPA, although this was not tested directly) were *abl, K-ras, yes, fps, src, bas, rel, ros, mos, erb-B, fms, erb-A,* and *raf.*

The two most striking aspects of *c-fos* induction are its rapidity and its transience. It is thus unlikely that any of the TPA-induced RNA and polypeptides reported in other studies were products of the *c-fos* gene, particularly since the *c-fos* 2.2-kb mRNA (which gives rise to a 55-kdalton translation product that is modified to give a stable 62-kdalton polypeptide) is not very stable in most cell types tested. The one previously identified gene product induced with comparable rapidity (that is, within 1 hr), was an unstable 50-kdalton polypeptide.[70] The methodologies employed in other work — pulse-labeling of protein or cDNA construction from total mRNA — necessarily gave up in temporal resolution and sensitivity what they gained in generality. In contrast, the "nuclear runoff" methodology employed by Greenberg and Ziff[96] is ideally suited for detection of gene products that are transiently expressed in relatively small amounts, and has the further advantage of measuring transcription activity directly. Important additional data should therefore be forthcoming from this type of analysis as the appropriate probes for other tumor promoter-responsive gene products become available.

Some insight into the mechanism of rapid transcriptional activation by tumor promoters has come from the observation that both *c-fos* and *c-myc* RNA could be induced in quiescent 3T3 cells by a 4-hr exposure to cycloheximide.[97] Cycloheximide, plus either high serum, PDGF, or TPA, caused superinduction of the RNAs in a number of different cell types well above levels caused by either treatment alone,[94,98,99,113] and a similar result has been obtained in a mouse endocrine tumor line, PC12, after inhibition of protein synthesis with anisomycin.[118] Even though the *c-fos* RNA induced in HL-60 cells by TPA was unusually stable, cycloheximide still caused superinduction.[114] This result makes it unlikely that the superinduction phenomenon is related to mRNA stability, rather than to mRNA production. Early adenovirus RNAs induced by TPA are also superinduced in the presence of cycloheximide.[35] A second parallel between the adenovirus case and induction of the *c-fos* and *c-myc* oncogenes is that the adenovirus Ela gene product is a positive regulator of transcription,[115-118] and this role has also been hypothesized for *myc.*[180] Because cycloheximide suppresses the transcription-delayed phenotype of adenovirus Ela mutants in productively infected HeLa cells[120] (Section III.B), it is possible that the same unstable cell-regulatory protein interacts with, or affects the expression of, a class of TPA-inducible genes that includes *fos, myc,* and the adenovirus early genes.

III. STIMULATION OF VIRUS GENE EXPRESSION BY TUMOR PROMOTERS

There is by now ample evidence that tumor promoters — in particular, TPA — can modulate virus gene expression in cells infected by a number of families of DNA and RNA viruses. Much of the impetus for this discovery, apart from a curiosity about how substances that regulate cell growth can interact with virus replication, has been the fact that members of a number of biologically very different virus groups can all act as carcinogens. It is therefore reasonable to expect that a study of the interaction of tumor promoters and virus gene expression will provide clues to both the mechanism of action of tumor promoters and also insight into the phenomenon of tumor promotion.

However, to understand the relevance of the virus model to tumor promotion, it is essential to distinguish between the virus as a carcinogen, with varied but specific mechanisms for inducing cell transformation, and the virus as a genetic entity, with a regulated developmental program of expression that is susceptible to modulation by factors that influence cellular physiology. Obviously, these two facets of the virus model may come together in important ways, such as the superinduction of a retrovirus and its associated oncogene (*v-onc*) by TPA,[121] or the discovery of mouse mammary tumor virus-related cell sequences induced by TPA in mouse lymphoid lines.[122] However, a direct induction of *v-onc* sequences by tumor promoters is not the only thing viruses have to tell us about the mechanism of action of tumor promoters. At present, our understanding of the regulation of virus gene expression far outstrips our understanding of analogous mechanisms in mammalian cells. Not only is it easier to identify, isolate, and manipulate viral genes; at present it is also easier to correlate in vitro structural information to in vivo function. As a result, it is possible to ask mechanistic questions of the virus model that may not yet be approachable in the uninfected cell.

A. Studies on Cells Transformed or Latently Infected by Viruses
1. Epstein-Barr Virus

Most studies of tumor-promoter action on viral gene expression have focused on cell lines that are either transformed or latently infected by viruses. For historical reasons unrelated to the study of tumor promotion, Epstein-Barr virus (EBV) was the first virus whose gene expression was shown to be affected by TPA. Lack of a permissive cell culture system for EBV[123] relegated studies of virus replication to spontaneous, or low-level, induction in certain transformed lines.[124-127] The discovery by zur Hausen and colleagues[128,129] that TPA could induce replication of the virus led to wide use of this promoter in EBV research, and consequent interest in the details of its effect on viral gene expression. At the present time, it is clear that cells containing EBV genomes are induced by TPA to synthesize early RNAs,[130-133] and that this effect is independent of viral or cellular DNA replication.[130,133,134] One of the major TPA-induced RNAs is transcribed from a region of the EBV genome that contains structural features thought to be analogous to the herpes simplex immediate early region.[132] Other viral RNA species are also induced in productively infected B-95 cells,[130,131,135] including some that may be specific to TPA-treated cells. In the nonproducer cell line P3HR-1, TPA induced the synthesis of six chromosome-associated polypeptides that were tentatively identified as viral in origin.[136]

Due to the complexity of the EBV genome, however, the details of its transcriptional regulation are still being worked out. It is therefore difficult at this point to assess the mechanistic significance of specific transcriptional changes caused by TPA. The induction of "immediate early" genes[132] might be sufficient to explain the overall stimulation of EBV replication, and would be consistent with observations of the effect of TPA on another DNA tumor virus, human adenovirus (Section III.B), and the rapid induction of specific cell genes (Section II).

2. Papovaviruses

In cells containing latent papovaviruses maintained in an episomal state, TPA has been found to induce DNA replication 1.4- to as much as 6-fold,[56,137] whereas no induction of integrated SV40 was observed in transformed cells.[137] This apparent specificity for episomal DNA, at least in the effect of TPA on replication of the HD strain of stump-tailed macaque virus, is reminiscent of the case of EBV, which is extrachromosomal in both producer and nonproducer lines. Induction by TPA of viral transcription and replication also occurred in mouse cells infected with bovine papilloma virus (BPV).[56] In these cells, infection by BPV is normally abortive; that is, no replication is observed, and after several passages the virus is lost from the cells. When infected cells were exposed to TPA, however, replication of BPV DNA was detected by Southern blot analysis 18 hr after infection, and persisted in high amounts long after it would otherwise have disappeared from uninfected cultures. The viral polyadenylated RNA species detected by Northern blot analysis after TPA treatment appeared to be the same as those in hamster cells transformed by BPV. The ability of TPA to stimulate BPV DNA synthesis and transcription was highly dependent on cell type.[56] No effect was observed in infected mouse kidney cells or in two lines of human fibroblasts; bovine cells showed line-dependent responses for DNA replication, but stimulation of transcription was either transient or absent; and rat-embryo fibroblasts showed only transient DNA synthesis. Lack of a clear response to TPA in at least several of these cases could not have been due to an intrinsic inability of the cell to respond to TPA, since effects of tumor promoters have been well-documented in rat and bovine cells. Thus, the differences in response were probably the result of differences in permissiveness for viral replication.

3. Retroviruses

The RNA tumor viruses are attractive subjects for the study of the effects of tumor promoters on viral gene expression because many of them are highly oncogenic, and because they carry analogs of mammalian oncogenes. Cells transformed by many of these viruses are persistently infected, in that they also produce newly synthesized virus particles while the cells continue to proliferate. A first attempt to relate the cellular effects of TPA to activation of an oncogene involved a study of cAMP-dependent, tyrosine-specific protein kinase activity in chick-embryo fibroblasts (CEF) transformed by the Schmidt-Ruppin strain of Rous sarcoma virus (RSV).[138] Since this enzyme is a product of both the viral oncogene *v-src* and its cellular analog *c-src*, induction of *c-src* by TPA would be a sufficient cause of cellular changes induced by TPA that mimic the transformed phenotype. However, no changes in cAMP-dependent protein kinase activity were observed in either normal or transformed cells after 3 days of TPA treatment. A modest (twofold) transient stimulation of this kinase activity was observed in untransformed CEF after 1 hr of exposure,[107] but TPA did not affect the viral-encoded kinase activity under conditions where it could be distinguished from the cellular enzyme. Finally, two-dimensional polyacrylamide gel analysis of polypeptides synthesized in CEF cells and in CEF cells transformed by RSV after 4, 8, and 24 hr of exposure to TPA, showed that phosphorylation of the putative cellular substrate for the *src* kinase was not significantly altered by TPA.[81] The conclusion that TPA did not induce *c-src* or stimulate *v-src* was corroborated by measurements of total cellular phosphotyrosine content, which did not change after exposure to TPA. Interestingly, a number of TPA-specific changes *were* observed, among them changes in the phosphorylation of other unidentified polypeptides.[81]

The effect of TPA on retrovirus gene expression depends upon the specific host-virus system studied. TPA increased the number of spleen focuses in Friend complex-infected mice, and also induced Friend leukemia virus and simian sarcoma virus release from producer cell lines, but the same promoting agent inhibited the production of endogenous virus by mitogen-treated mouse cell cultures.[139] On the other hand, TPA alone, or in combination with iododeoxyuridine (IUdR), induced murine xenotropic type-C retroviruses,[140] and enhanced production of murine leukemia virus.[141] TPA enhanced Mason-Pfizer monkey virus replication in human embryonic kidney cells, but not in a persistently infected human cell line.[142]

Mouse mammary tumor virus (MMTV) is an interesting example of a retrovirus that may contain genetic sequences which confer a specific responsiveness to tumor promoters, as well as to other agents that regulate cellular gene activity. In persistently infected mouse mammary tumor cells, both TPA and dexamethasone separately stimulated MMTV RNA synthesis and virus production.[121] These agents act synergistically, however, together they increased virus RNA synthesis further by a factor of five. This effect was specific for phorbol esters with tumor-promoting activity (and also for MMTV) since induction of type-C endogenous virus was not detected in the same cells. It is unlikely that the same viral sequences that control response to corticosteroids also define a target for regulation by TPA. The mechanisms of genetic regulation by corticosteroids and peptide growth hormones are known to be quite different, and available evidence suggests that regulation of gene expression by peptide growth hormones and TPA have many common features (Section II.C).[143-149] In any event, corticosteroid synergism with tumor promoters is highly atypical. Other than the stimulation of MMTV transcription and the induction of collagenase in rabbit synovial fibroblasts,[79,80] corticosteroids have usually been found to antagonize the effects of tumor promoters in both transformation[150,151] and viral replication.[152]

A recent report on the induction of MMTV-like sequences in mouse lymphocytes by TPA suggests that homologous sequences may be targets of the response of normal cells to tumor promoters.[121] cDNA libraries were prepared from the murine leukemic cell line EL-4 and screened by differential hybridization to identify TPA-inducible sequences. Of 17 clones identified as consistently inducible, 6 were related in sequence to MMTV. This abundant inducible sequence included part of the *env* gene and the right long terminal repeat (LTR) of MMTV, but the nucleotide sequence of the clone was substantially divergent from the sequence of MMTV provirus. Interestingly, two out of five steroid-binding sites were present, intact in the LTR region of the cloned sequence. RNA containing the MMTV sequence was induced by TPA in normal spleen cells from Balb/c and C57Bl/6 mice, as well as in EL-4 cells, although the response of the transformed line to TPA was more intense than in the normal cells.

B. Studies on Acutely Infected Cells
1. Rationale
Relatively little work has involved the effect of tumor promoters on viral gene expression during the initial stages of infection, whether in lytic (productive) or transforming (abortive or productive) systems. Among the herpes viruses, TPA has been shown to stimulate virus polypeptide synthesis of *Herpes saimari*,[129] but to have no detectable effect on the replication of simian varicella virus.[153] The short-term effects of TPA and other phorbol esters on human adenovirus include acceleration of the replicative cycle,[34] and induction of early transcription.[35] Such studies are important for two reasons: (1) that the use of viruses to arrive at an understanding of the role of TPA as a promoter of transformation must ultimately focuses on the early stages of infection rather than on events occurring in a cell that has already been transformed by the virus; and (2) the genetic program of certain viruses in lytically infected cells is now understood in some detail. This is particularly true of human adenovirus,[154] and is a prerequisite for in vivo and in vitro studies of mechanism.

2. Regulation of Adenovirus Gene Expression
Early adenovirus transcription is under the control of at least two virus genes: a product of region Ela (0 to 4.5 map units on a 100-unit scale) which facilitates early transcription[115,117] and the 72-kdalton encoded by region E2a (61 to 75 map units) which lowers the steady-state level of early viral RNAs by acting on both transcription[155-157] and RNA stability.[118,158]

The mechanism of Ela action is under active invetigation. Present evidence indicates that an Ela gene product directly or indirectly facilitates transcription from early viral promoters, possibly by inactivating a cell-encoded repressor.[117,120,159] Primary transcripts from the Ela region are processed early in infection to give 12s and 13s mRNAs which differ in splicing pattern.[154] The regulatory product is probably synthesized from the 13s species because some virus mutations that delay early transcription, such as hrl, map in the intron of the 12s mRNA.[160,161] Stimulation of early adenovirus transcription by Ela is specific, because it depends upon DNA sequences 5′ to the transcriptional starts of the early genes.[116] The curious finding that, in sequential double infections with different adenovirus mutants, Ela appears to act only in *cis* with the genome that encodes it,[162] could be explained by the formation of a structural complex between the infecting viral genome, the Ela product, and cell constituents. The hypothesis that the nuclear matrix is involved in this complex is supported by the finding that the regulatory Ela polypeptide is localized on this structure.[163] These disparate results can be organized into a tentative model of Ela action as follows: early adenovirus transcription may require formation of a transcriptional complex that involves the nuclear matrix proteins; formation of the complex is facilitated by the Ela regulatory protein, but occurs slowly in its absence, depends on specific viral sequences, and is inhibited by a functionally unstable cellular protein. One of the possible mechanisms of Ela action might be neutralization of this putative cellular inhibitor.

3. Laboratory Investigations

a. Acceleration of Adenovirus Gene Expression by TPA

Carter et al.[34,35] have been investigating the effect of phorbol ester tumor promoters, and in particular of TPA, on the regulation of human type-5 adenovirus gene expression during productive infection of HeLa cells. Contributions from their laboratory to a collaborative study[34] established that the acceleration of adenovirus replication by TPA could be detected during the first few hours after infection by measuring the appearance of viral mRNA in the cytoplasm. These measurements were done by adding TPA to infected-cell monolayers 1 hr after virus adsorption, incubating at 33°C, and labeling with ^{3}H-uridine for 2-hr periods during the first 20 hr of infection. Cytoplasmic RNA was poly(A)-selected, and the amount of viral RNA from early regions of the genome in this fraction was determined by quantitative filter hybridization. Messenger RNA from all early regions appeared ahead of schedule, and more RNA hybridizing to the E3 region was consistently detected in TPA-treated cells, compared to controls. Carter et al. concluded from these results that the action of TPA was rapid, and that the effect on viral mRNA production was probably sufficient to explain the observed acceleration of virus replication.

The investigators have also quantitated the amount of cytoplasmic viral RNA in TPA-treated cells by dot-blotting (Figure 1). TPA clearly accelerated the appearance and accumulation of viral RNA in HeLa cells, but not in MRC-5, a line of diploid human fibroblasts. This result is consistent with the observation of others that primary human cells and untransformed human cell lines are refractory to many of the usual effects of TPA,[28,82] whereas transformed human cells, such as HeLa, are responsive.[59,89]

b. In Vivo Studies of the Effect of TPA on Transcription

Carter et al. next determined that the increase in cytoplasmic viral RNA in TPA-treated cells at early times after infection was the result of an earlier transcriptional start, rather than a posttranscriptional effect such as transport or differential stability. In the first set of experiments, the relative rate of transcription of various early regions

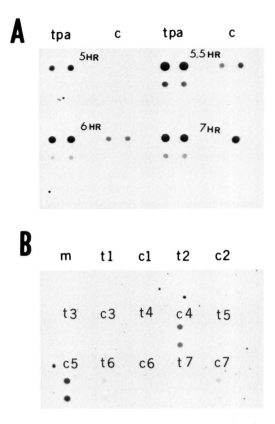

FIGURE 1. Effect of TPA on the cytoplasmic concentration of RNA from early-region E3 in Ad5-infected human cells. Panel A: Duplicate samples of RNA from HeLa cells were spotted in three successive fivefold dilutions on nitrocellulose paper and hybridized to nick-translated E3 probe. At each time point, samples were compared from TPA-treated (tpa) and control (c) cells. Panel B: Duplicate samples from Ad5-infected MRC-5 cells were spotted and hybridized as in Panel A, except that no dilutions were used. The numbers refer to the time, in hours postinfection, at which the samples were taken.

was measured by pulse-labeling TPA-treated and control cells for 5 min, and filter hybridization of the purified RNA.[35] Again, a pronounced acceleration was observed in the appearance of labeled viral RNA from all early regions, strongly implicating transcription as an early target of TPA action (Figure 2). Although the accleration of 2 hr appears small in relationship to the 24- to 36-hr replicative cycle of Ad5, it amounts to a *halving* of the period between infection and first detection of viral transcription. It is also possible to conclude from the pulse-labeling data that the transient overproduction of E3 RNA observed after TPA treatment could be explained by a slightly prolonged and stimulated rate of E3 transcription.

An important point in the interpretation of subsequent data is that the main, consistent effect of TPA on Ad5 gene expression is to accelerate the transcriptional program, rather than to stimulate the maximal transcription rate. Fixed-time comparisons

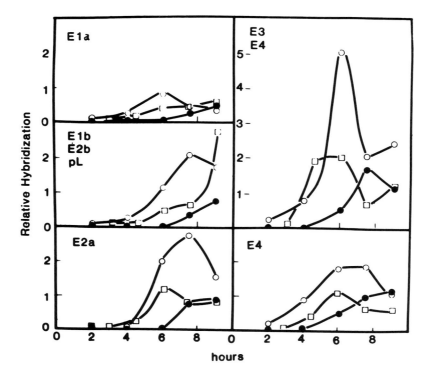

FIGURE 2. Rate of Ad5 early-region transcription in HeLa cells treated with 25 μg/ mℓ cycloheximide (closed circles), 100 ng/mℓ TPA (open squares), or both (open circles).

of transcription rate, however, will reflect this earlier onset of transcription in TPA-treated cells as an enhanced rate. Carter et al. have used this fixed-time assay to screen a number of chemical agents and conditions for their effects on the phenomenon at hand (see below). They also determined by this means that only phorbol esters with tumor-promoting activity on mouse skin were able to accelerate viral transcription (Table 3).

Figure 2 also contains data obtained when cycloheximide was added to the infected HeLa cells at the same time as TPA. Carter et al. found that inhibition of protein synthesis did not prevent the acceleration of the onset of viral RNA synthesis by TPA, and concluded that a TPA-induced protein is not responsible for early induction of early viral RNA. Somewhat surprisingly, the maximal rate of all early viral transcription was increased by cycloheximide, but only in TPA-treated cells. This superinduction may be analogous to the superinduction of several cell genes by TPA in cycloheximide-treated cells (Section II.C).[94,98,99,112,113] They proposed that a cell protein, the synthesis or activity of which was inhibited by cycloheximide, had become, in TPA-treated cells, a limiting factor on the observed rate of viral transcription.

It is possible that an accelerated onset of viral transcription after infection of permissive cells could result from earlier arrival of viral DNA in the nucleus. Carter et al. tested this possibility by measuring the association of radiolabeled virion DNA with the nucleus during the first 8 hr after virus adsorption.[35] The movement of viral DNA to the nuclear fraction followed linear kinetics and was not altered by TPA. This experimental procedure did not distinguish between functional and physical association of the viral DNA with the cell nucleus, thus, it is still possible that TPA facilitates the

Table 3
EFFECT OF TPA AND
RELATED COMPOUNDS ON
AD5 TRANSCRIPTION AT 7 HR
POSTINFECTION

	Relative hybridization[a]	
Addition	Experiment 1	Experiment 2
DMSO	(1.0)	(1.0)
TPA	1.7	3.6
PDD[b]	1.5	3.6
4-α-PDD	1.3	1.3
Phorbol	0.9	1.3

[a]   HeLa monolayers were infected for 1 hr
and then exposed to drug or solvent
(DMSO) for 6 hr before a 10-min pulse-
labeling with ^{3}H-uridine. Viral RNA synthesis was determined by dividing the cpm
hybridized to filters containing whole
viral DNA by the total cpm input, and
was then normalized to the control
(DMSO-treated) value for each experiment.

[b]   PDD = phorbol-12,13-didecanoate.

formation of a functional complex within the nucleus. In any event, their results are consistent with the hypothesis that TPA does not accelerate virus gene expression by increasing the total number of DNA templates potentially available for transcription.

In assessing the speed with which TPA can exert its effect on adenovirus gene expression during lytic infection, Carter et al. were faced with a complex situation. Virus gene expression, as part of a developmental program, changes with time after infection and depends upon prior regulatory events. Thus, TPA added at various times during this process is liable to exert different effects on the expression of a given gene, depending upon when the promoter is added; this proved to be the case (Figure 3).[164] HeLa cells growing in monolayer were infected with Ad5 for 6 hr, at which time radiolabeled uridine was added for 5 min and the radioactivity of viral RNA analyzed by filter hybridization. TPA was added at different times to replicate cultures during the incubation period, up to and including the 5 min of labeling. Thus, time on the abscissa in Figure 3 represents hours of exposure to TPA, rather than time after infection. However, the duration of exposure is also inversely related to the time at which TPA was added after infection. The results of three experiments are shown. Although there was considerable quantitative variability in data, several conclusions appear warranted. First, exposure to TPA for as little as 5 min (that is, during the labeling period at 6 hr *after* infection) resulted in a reproducible but variable increase in the rate of Ad5 transcription from all early regions. Second, different patterns of TPA stimulation were apparent for different early regions. These can be interpreted consistently when the data are viewed not as a function of the length of exposure to TPA, but rather as a function of the time at which TPA was added in relationship to the transcriptional program of the virus. For example, stimulation of transcription from E3 at 6 hr postinfection ranged from 1.6-fold to more than 4-fold, but appeared to be independent of the time of TPA addition. E4 transcription was increased only if the promoter was added during the last 2 hr before labeling, whereas the rate of E2a transcrip-

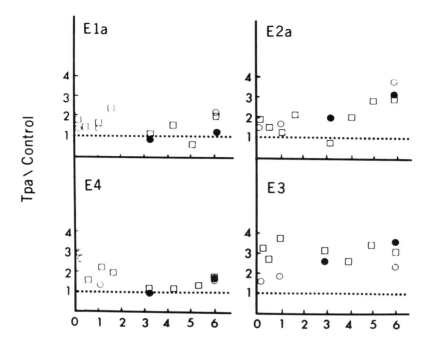

FIGURE 3.   Effect of length of exposure to TPA on rate of Ad5 early transcription at 6 hr postinfection.

tion appeared to be inversely related to the time after infection at which TPA was added. E4 is normally expressed late in the early phase of infection, starting at about the time when RNA was labeled in this experiment; the onset of E2a expression precedes that of E4, and decreases at the time when E4 transcription is maximal. E3 behaves much like E2a during normal infection. Thus, the results are consistent with the hypothesis that the effect of TPA is not to stimulate transcription of most early genes directly, but instead to accelerate the transcriptional program of the virus. The possible exception to this pattern occurs in the E3 region, where the preferential stimulation of E3 transcription[34,35] may reflect a difference in the way E3 is regulated, compared to other early genes.

Because of the rapidity with which TPA was able to exert its effects on Ad5 transcription, Carter et al. were also interested in determining whether continuous exposure to TPA was required for stimulation of transcription, or whether prior exposure was sufficient. In two separate experiments, the overall rate of viral transcription was measured by hybridization at 3 or 6 hr after infection, and TPA was added at different and varying lengths of time.[164] Prior to infection, 6 hr of TPA exposure, followed by removal of the promoter, caused the same magnitude of effect as when TPA was present continuously. It was concluded that the TPA-induced alterations in cell physiology that lead to altered gene activity persist for at least 6 hr in HeLa cells, and do not require the continuous presence of TPA in the medium. In these experiments Carter et al. did not measure TPA bound to the cell membrane; thus, it is possible that a tightly bound promoter could continue to exert its effects over a 6-hr period.

In attempting to assess the possible mechanisms by which a tumor promoter acting at the cell membrane could transduce a regulatory signal to the nucleus within a matter of minutes, the investigators[32,33] were struck by the observation that rapid cytoskeletal changes occur in cells exposed to TPA. These changes involve phosphorylation of cytoskeletal proteins; binding of TPA to the cell membrane is known to activate a specific

Table 4

EFFECT OF ANTITUMOR DRUGS ON TPA
STIMULATION OF AD5 TRANSCRIPTION

		% Viral RNA[b]	
Addition[a]	Experiment	No TPA	+ TPA
None	1	.11	.14
Colchicine	1	.20	.06
Podophyllotoxin	1	.07	.005
Vinblastine	1	.03	.03
Cytochalasin B	1	.02	.08
None	2	.05	.16
Taxol	2	.05	.14

[a]   DMSO (solvent control), TPA, and drug +/− TPA were
added 1 hr postinfection, and RNA was labeled for 1 hr with
^{3}H-uridine starting at 4.4 hr.

[b]   % of total radioactivity hybridized to all early regions of the
Ad5 genome.

protein kinase.[147] Therefore, it was possible that drugs which interfere with various components of the cytoskeletal framework could also prevent the stimulation of Ad5 gene expression by TPA.[164] HeLa monolayers were infected with Ad5, and 1 hr later TPA was added with or without one of the following drugs: colchicine, vinblastine, podophyllotoxin, cytochalasin B, or Taxol. The overall rate of Ad5 transcription was measured at 5.5 hr, as described previously. Interpretation of the data is complicated by the possible effects of the drugs alone on viral gene expression, thus, transcription was also measured in the presence of the drugs alone. The results of two experiments are shown in Table 4. Although vinblastine and cytochalasin B both inhibited viral gene expression, they did not cause a reduction in overall incorporation of radiolabeled uridine, implying that these two agents interfered specifically with the process of viral infection. A stimulation of viral transcription by TPA occurred in cells treated with either cytochalasin B or taxol, but not colchicine, podophyllotoxin, or vinblastine, when compared to the rate observed in the presence of the cytoskeleton-acting drug alone. The fact that these latter three drugs are known to disrupt microtubular structure[167] (whereas cytochalasin B disrupts microfilaments[165] and taxol stabilizes microtubules)[166] suggests that an integral, functioning microtubular system is needed for the effect of TPA on Ad5 transcription.

c. Interaction of TPA with Viral Gene Products

The lack of requirement for new protein synthesis to obtain the acceleration of viral transcription by TPA predicted that mutants defective in early viral functions should respond to TPA in the same way as wild-type (wt) virus. When HeLa cells were infected with temperature-sensitive mutants in E2a (H5 *ts*125) or E2b (H5 *ts*149) at the nonpermissive temperature, TPA still accelerated the onset of transcription from all early regions by 1 to 2 hr.[35]

The effect of TPA on viral gene expression in cells infected by Ela mutants was also of interest, however in the absence of protein synthesis inhibitors, early transcription from these mutant genomes is much delayed. HeLa cells were therefore infected with a low multiplicity of either the Ad5 mutant hrl or wild-type (wt) virus, exposed to TPA or solvent continuously from 1 to 6 hr after infection, lysed, and the polyadenylated cytoplasmic RNA analyzed for virus sequences by "Northern" blot analysis. Figure 4

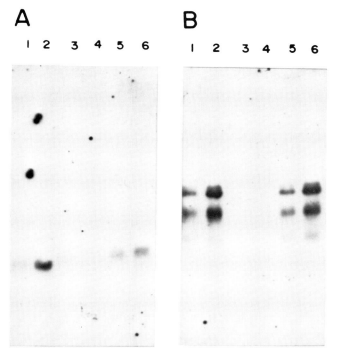

FIGURE 4. Effect of TPA on cytoplasmic polyadenylated RNA species in HeLa cells infected by the Ela mutant, hrl. Panel A: Northern blot probed with Ela. Panel B: Northern blot probed with E3. Lanes 1 and 2: RNA from wt-infected cells; lanes 3 and 4: hrl RNA from control cells; lanes 5 and 6, hrl RNA from TPA-treated cells.

shows autoradiograms of two blots, one hybridized to probe for the Ela region, and the other to probe for the E3 region. For comparison, polyadenylated RNA from wt-infected cells was run in lanes 1 and 2 on both panels. Without TPA, no E3 mRNA was detected in hrl-infected cells (lanes B3 and B4). However, all E3 RNA species observed in wt-infected cells (lanes 1 and 2) were also observed in hrl-infected cells treated with TPA and were present in amounts roughly equal to those in wt infection. A small amount of Ela mRNA was detected in control hrl-infected cells treated with DMSO (lanes A3 and A4), and this too was increased in amount by exposure of the cells to TPA (lanes A5 and A6). Quantitative filter hybridization of pulse-labeled RNA from hrl-infected cells was consistent with the Northern blot analysis, and showed that transcription from all early regions was restored by TPA.[35]

From the above-mentioned experiments with hrl, Carter et al. concluded that TPA can either replace the Ela transcriptional function, or allow the truncated Ela polypeptide produced in hrl-infected cells[168] to perform its transcriptional function normally. Interestingly, Carter et al. also found that TPA did not restore the ability of hrl to replicate in HeLa cells which are nonpermissive for this mutant due to the absence of an intact Ela gene. This result suggests either that TPA does not completely substitute for the Ela regulatory product, or that this product has multiple functions, only one of which can be circumvented by TPA. At present investigators cannot distinguish between these possibilities. One approach would be to test the effect of TPA on viral transcription in other Ela mutants lacking some or all of the regulatory protein. These experiments are now in progress.

d. Viral Transcription in Isolated Nuclei

Another approach to measuring transcription activity during an in vivo experiment is to isolate nuclei and measure their ability to incorporate radiolabeled uridine triphosphate (UTP) in vitro by transcription of endogenous template DNA. In one type of preparation, RNA polymerase is not able to initiate transcription; incorporation of UTP in this system reflects the extension of nascent RNA chains, and therefore measures the number and activity of transcription complexes present in the nuclei at the time of isolation.[169,170] In this case, transcription ceases after 20 to 30 min, presumably when all nascent RNA molecules have been completed. A second type of preparation allows *de novo* initiation or reinitiation of RNA polymerase II, resulting in prolonged transcription over 1 to 2 hr or more.[171,172] Incorporation of labeled UTP in this system reflects the ability of RNA polymerase II to bind productively to endogenous promoters under *in vitro* conditions.

Carter et al. have used both types of isolated nuclear systems to study the effect of TPA on Ad5 transcription. Their results can be summarized as follows:[35,164]

1. Transcription of viral DNA is two to three times more active in "noninitiating" nuclei isolated from TPA-treated cells than from controls at the latest time when in vivo transcription is maximally different in the two conditions (6 hr postinfection, 5 hr after TPA addition); aggregate transcription of other sequences (total incorporation of UTP) in nuclei isolated from TPA-treated cells was unchanged.
2. Prolonged transcription in "initiating" nuclei from TPA-treated cells produced three to seven times as much viral RNA as similar preparations from control cells; these differences were comparable to those obtained in parallel experiments in which viral RNA was pulse-labeled in vivo.
3. TPA added directly to isolated nuclear preparations had no effect on the rate of viral transcription.
4. Zakeri and Carter[183] did not detect an increased chemical stability of labeled virus RNA synthesized in vitro by nuclei from TPA-treated cells.

These results allow a number of conclusions about the mechanism of TPA action. First, interaction of TPA with an intact cell, or, minimally, with extranuclear components, is required for its effect on transcription. Second, the results imply that either more RNA polymerase II is available to transcribe specifically viral DNA in TPA-treated cells, or that the polymerase in these cells is better able to engage in transcription from early viral promoters. This latter possibility could result from either an activation of the RNA polymerase molecule (or its associated factors), or from an alteration of the viral template in TPA-treated cells. These models can best be experimentally distinguished from each other in purified, reconstructed systems, in which it is possible to manipulate the enzyme and template independently. The laboratory of the investigators is now pursuing this line of investigation.

e. Transcription in Soluble Whole-Cell Extracts

Manley et al.[173-176] are using soluble whole-cell extracts isolated from TPA-treated and control HeLa cells to transcribe Ad5 DNA and cloned fragments of Ad5 or Ad2 DNA that contain early promoters. In preliminary, unpublished, experiments using extracts from Ad5-infected cells to transcribe whole-viral DNA or mixtures of restriction endonuclease-generated fragments of whole-viral DNA, extracts from TPA-treated cells consistently transcribed viral templates more actively than extracts from untreated cells, as determined by total incorporation of UTP into macromolecular product. This difference was not observed when calf thymus DNA was used as template. Quantitative analysis by filter hybridization of the in vitro products from transcription of adenovirus DNA confirmed that TPA extracts were more active on all regions of the DNA. This enhancement was most pronounced at low concentrations of template, and occasionally could not be seen at DNA inputs greater than 150 μg/mℓ. Similar results were obtained with three different paired extract preparations (TPA and control), and one pair of extracts from uninfected cells. These, and all subsequent extracts, were prepared simultaneously from the same batch of cells treated with TPA or solvent in order to minimize the effect of artifacts that might be introduced during the preparation of the extracts.

"Runoff transcription" from cloned viral DNA containing early promoters (and cleaved enzymatically at a site downstream from the nucleotide corresponding to the 5′ end of the primary transcript) has confirmed that soluble extracts from TPA-treated cells are more active on early virus genes than are extracts from control cells. Furthermore, the effect appears to be specific, at least for some early genes, since both extracts transcribe the adenovirus major late promoter equally well. An example of recent data is shown in Figure 5. In a typical experiment several concentrations of DNA are used because of the sensitivity of transcription rate in vitro (and the TPA effect) to template concentration. After transcription for a fixed period, usually 60 min, the labeled RNA is purified and analyzed by denaturing agarose gel electrophoresis and autoradiography. Promoter-specific transcripts are recognized by their mobilities relative to size standards. Quantitative data were obtained either by scanning the autoradiograph with a densitometer, or by excising the bands from the gel and determining their content of radiolabel by scintillation spectrometry.

Figure 5 shows the dependence of transcription rate from the Ela promoter on DNA concentration, and also the difference in activity between TPA and control extracts. The major runoff products from this promoter include in this case two bands with approximate molecular sizes of 740 and 820 bp. These probably correspond to initiation at the promoter utilized in vivo (740-bp runoff), as well as at a site upstream from this promoter that is recognized by RNA polymerase only in vitro.[173] Synthesis of runoff products was inhibited by α amanitin at 1 μg/mℓ, indicating that the enzyme being assayed was RNA polymerase II.[164]

Figure 6, which compares runoff transcription from the Ela and major late virus promoters at a series of DNA concentrations, illustrates the specificity of the TPA effect for the Ela early promoter, but not for the major late promoter. Quantitation of the labeled transcripts by excision from the gel and determination of radioactivity showed that polymerase from TPA-treated cells was more active in transcribing the Ela promoter than the major late promoter.

There is now preliminary evidence, from experiments in which extracts from TPA-treated and control cells were mixed, that the difference in Ela transcription may be caused by an inhibitor in the control extracts. A series of reactions were carried out at a fixed DNA concentration, comparing the activities of extracts singly and in equal mixtures containing increasing amounts of total protein (Figure 7). At each concentration of extract protein, the TPA extract was more active than the control, but a mixture of the two abolished this enhanced activity.

One important conclusion that can be drawn from these in vitro studies is that the effect of TPA on adenovirus gene expression does not involve alteration of the viral chromatin, but rather a change in the cellular environment that affects either DNA structure or the RNA polymerase itself. If a similar mechanism was responsible for the stimulation of cell gene expression by TPA, it should also be possible to observe this effect in soluble extracts containing cloned promoters from such TPA-responsive genes.

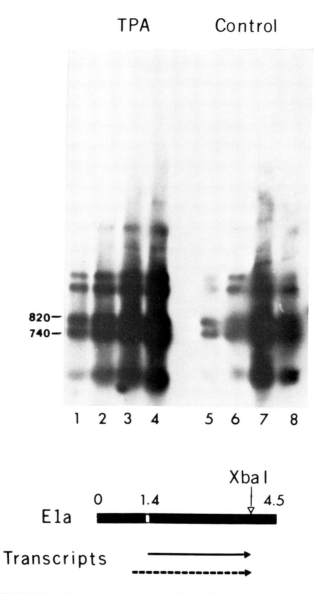

FIGURE 5.   Runoff transcription of Ela DNA by soluble whole-cell extracts from TPA-treated and control cells. Cloned DNA from the leftmost 4.5% of the Ad5 genome was cut with XbaI and transcribed in reactions containing increasing amounts of DNA. Lanes 1 and 5: 30 μg/mℓ; lanes 2 and 6: 40 μg/mℓ; lanes 3 and 7: 50 μg/mℓ; lanes 4 and 8: 60 μg/mℓ.

Much additional work needs to be done to characterize the stimulation of in vitro transcription by TPA. The many questions to be answered include whether the effect is specific for all adenovirus early promoters; whether transcription from other viral or cellular promoters is affected in the same way; and whether the stimulation of transcription by TPA results from a direct effect on the RNA polymerase or on its regulatory factors. Answers to these questions may help to elucidate a key step in the mechanism of tumor-promoter action on gene expression.

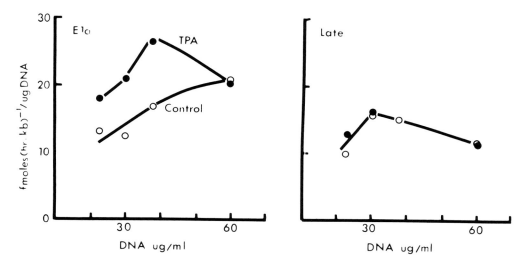

FIGURE 6. Runoff transcription from the Ela and major late promoters. Transcripts were quantitated by excision from the gel and scintillation counting. The values were then normalized for length of the runoff product and the concentration of template DNA.

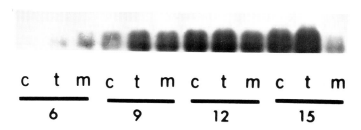

FIGURE 7. Effect of extract mixing on transcription of Ela DNA. c = control, t = TPA, m = equal mixture of control and TPA extracts. Total concentration of extract protein in mg/mℓ is indicated below each set of three reactions.

IV. SUMMARY AND CONCLUSIONS

The expression of a number of cell genes is modulated by exposure to tumor promoters — A common heuristic framework for studying the phenomenon of tumor promotion has been the resemblance between the transformed phenotype and many of the morphologic and biochemical changes caused by exposure of untransformed cells to tumor-promoting agents. For example, synthesis of several excreted glycoproteins, of plasminogen activator, and of the enzymes of polyamine biosynthesis is increased in both transformed and "promoted" cells, whereas the synthesis of another glycoprotein is decreased in both cell types. Among the cellular proto-oncogenes, transcription of *c-fos* and *c-myc* is stimulated rapidly by tumor promoters in a variety of cells from different species. The activation of *c-myc* is widely associated with the transformed phenotype. Decreased expression of both *c-myc* and *c-myb* after TPA treatment of thyroid and hematopoetic tumor cells correlates with cessation of proliferation. Certain oncogenes such as *Ha-ras* have been shown to act secondarily to oncogenes of the *c-myc* class during transformation in vitro, and alone are unable to transform certain cells in culture. Since *Ha-ras* can thus be thought of as an oncogene analog of a tumor promoter, it would be interesting to determine whether genes of this class are activated by phorbol esters. This has not yet been tested directly, although PDGF, serum, and fibroblast growth factor, which act like TPA in stimulating *c-fos* and *c-myc* transcription in 3T3 cells, do not increase expression of *K-ras* in these cells.

The effects of tumor promoters on gene expression are dependent upon cell type — This dependence generally reflects commitment of the cell to a proliferative or a differentiative pathway. Untransformed cells are characteristically encouraged by tumor promoters to proliferate, with concomitant expression of genes required for, or accompanying, cell division. Certain malignant cells, on the other hand, and possibly those normal cells that are committed to differentiate, often respond to tumor promoters in the opposite way, expressing differentiation-specific genes appropriate to the particular cell (such as β globin, calcitonin, prolactin, collagenase, keratins, and epidermal transglutaminase) and shutting off expression of some proto-oncogenes.

The modulation of gene expression by tumor promoters is mediated by a rapid effect on transcription — Induction of gene products by these agents is typically sensitive to actinomycin D and is accompanied by an increased level of translatable mRNA. Rapid increases in mRNA for ODC, plasminogen activator, calcitonin, prolactin, and several glycoproteins have been documented by cell-free translation of polyadenylated RNA isolated within 8 hr after exposure to TPA, and in some cases within 2 hr. In cases where nucleic acid probes have been available, TPA has been shown to stimulate transcription; these include cellular proto-oncogenes, prolactin, β actin, MMTV-related sequences, and early genes from both EBV and human adenovirus. Thus it is likely that an initial effect of tumor promoters, at least those of the phorbol ester type, is to activate transcription at a limited number of sites on cell and virus genomes. These sites may share structural homologies within a set of related genes, such as the adenovirus early genes or the putative gene families related to *c-fos*, prolactin, or MMTV; in each of these cases, there is indirect or suggestive evidence for the existence of homologous sequences which may include regulatory signals. It is also possible that there are common regulatory sequences which are shared by all genes that are rapidly inducible by tumor promoters. The only direct evidence relating nucleic acid sequence to tumor-promoter inducibility comes from the rat prolactin gene, in which sequences 5′ to the genetic promoter confer the property of inducibility by both TPA and EGF to genes that are normally not responsive to these agents. Additional information should be forthcoming from transient expression assays using cloned tumor promoter-responsive genes, or from in vitro transcription of DNA carrying potential regulatory sequences.

A common feature of the induction of gene expression by TPA is that inhibitors of protein synthesis not only fail to prevent enhanced transcription of many target genes, but often act synergistically with TPA to cause their superinduction. This result is consistent with the existence of a cellular repressor of TPA-inducible genes that must be continuously synthesized in order to exert its effects. The necessity for continued synthesis could imply either chemical or functional instability. Functional instability could result from a stoichiometric or irreversible participation in formation of transcription complexes, for example. In this case, pulse-chase experiments may fail to identify such a regulatory molecule. The superinduction phenomenon further implies that TPA can activate transcription of repressed genes by a mechanism that does not involve inactivation of the putative repressor. Results from in vitro transcription of adenovirus early genes by extracts from TPA-treated cells imply that at least one component of the induction of gene expression by phorbol esters involves a modification of RNA polymerase II specificity. This activation could occur by various mechanisms including loss of an inhibitor, modification of a regulatory factor, or alteration of the polymerase molecule itself. Whatever the mechanism, it must be rapid, because effects of TPA on transcription of both viral and cell genes are seen as early as 5 min after binding to receptors on the cell surface.

The biochemical pathway of the regulatory signal is largely unknown — The rapidity of TPA action on gene expression, like that of the peptide growth hormones, implies that this signal is communicated indirectly from the cell surface to the nucleus without involving endocytosis of the promoter and its receptor. Although a detailed discussion of this aspect of tumor-promoter action is beyond the scope of this chapter, it is pertinent to mention several points here. The receptor for phorbol ester tumor promoters has been characterized as a serine-specific, phospholipid-stimulated, calcium-activated, and cyclic AMP-independent protein kinase.[146,147] Targets for this kinase include the receptor for EGF, which is itself a tyrosine-specific, cyclic AMP-dependent protein kinase.[145,146,148,149] Protein phosphorylation may thus play a key role in transducing the growth-regulatory signals of both tumor promoters and peptide growth hormones, which also share the ability to induce certain cell genes. In this context, it may be significant that thyrotropin-releasing hormone causes rapid phosphorylation of several nuclear proteins,[100] and shares with TPA the ability to induce prolactin transcription. Other similarities between peptide growth hormones and phorbol ester tumor promoters include the rapid induction of *c-fos*, β actin, and *c-myc* genes in several mouse cell lines. The cytoskeletal network may play a role in signal transduction, because drugs that interfere with microtubular assembly or function also prevent induction of several genes by TPA. However, it is possible that these drugs interfere with TPA action by some mechanism unrelated to their effects on microtubules.

In summary, it is now possible to draw on information from many laboratories, using disparate experimental systems to construct the outline of a model for the regulation of gene expression by tumor promoters.

1. The promoter binds to a receptor on the cell surface, modulating the activity of one or more protein kinases.
2. Altered kinase activity changes the pattern of phosphorylation of cell proteins involved either in transducing the regulatory signal to the nucleus (e.g., microtubules or soluble proteins), or in regulating transcription directly, or both.
3. Altered nuclear proteins (phosphorylated?) allow transcription of a set of genes that includes some or all of those that are activated by certain polypeptide growth hormones; some of these nuclear regulatory factors are likely to be directly involved in the specificity of RNA polymerase II, rather than in the structure of chromatin, although chromatin changes may play an additional role.
4. Induction of target genes leads to further, secondary changes in gene expression that include both positive and negative regulation.
6. These changes lead ultimately to the survival and proliferation of initiated cells, which might otherwise be triggered in response to biochemical events surrounding initiation to enter an apoptotic pathway leading to cell death.

ACKNOWLEDGMENTS

The author wishes to thank Paul Fisher for stimulating his interest in tumor promotion, Gerhard Sauer and Ed Ziff for permission to quote unpublished results, Lee Babiss for both cloned DNA fragments and advice, and Nezrine Batturay and Richard Lockshin for helpful suggestions concerning the manuscript. Some of the data shown in the chapter was the work of Zahra Zakeri, Mary Waldron, and Luis Alejo in the laboratory of the author. The work from the author's laboratory, as well as the writing of this chapter, was supported in part by grants CA15757 and CA37761 to T. H. Carter from the National Institutes of Health.

REFERENCES

1. Van Duuren, B. L., Tumor-promoting agents in two-stage carcinogenesis, *Prog. Exp. Tumor Res.,* 11, 31, 1969.
2. Berenblum, I., Sequential aspects of chemical carcinogenesis: skin, in *Cancer, A Comprehensive Treatise,* Vol. 1, Becker, F. F., Ed., Plenum Press, New York, 1975, 323.
3. Sivak, A. and Van Duuren, B. L., RNA synthesis induction in cell culture by a tumor promoter, *Cancer Res.,* 30, 1203, 1970.
4. Scribner, J. D. and Boutwell, R. K., Inflamation and tumor promotion: selective protein induction in mouse skin by tumor promoters, *Eur. J. Cancer,* 8, 617, 1972.
5. Bhisey, R. A., Ramchandani, A. G., and Sirsat, S. M., Effects of 12-o-tetradecanoylphorbol-13-acetate on the incorporation of labeled precursors into RNA, DNA and protein in epidermis, dermis, and subcutis from precancerous mouse skin with reference to enhanced tumorigenesis, *Carcinogenesis,* 5, 135, 1984.
6. Balmain, A., The synthesis of specific proteins in adult mouse epidermis during phases of proliferation and differentiation induced by the tumor promoter TPA, and in basal and differentiating layers of neonatal mouse epidermis, *J. Invest. Dermatol.,* 67, 246, 1976.
7. Balmain, A., Alonso, A., and Fisher, J., Histone phosphorylation, DNA and RNA synthesis during phases of proliferation and differentiation induced in mouse epidermis by the tumor promoter 12-o-tetradecanoyl-phorbol-13-acetate, *Cancer Res.,* 37, 1548, 1977.
8. Balmain, A., Synthesis of specific proteins in mouse epidermis after treatment with the tumor promoter TPA, in *Carcinogenesis,* Vol. 2, Slaga, T. J., Sivak, A., and Boutwell, R. K., Eds., Raven Press, New York, 1978, 153.
9. Balmain, A., Loehren, D., Fisher, J., and Alonso, A., Protein synthesis during fetal development of mouse epidermis. I. The appearance of histidine-rich protein, *Dev. Biol.,* 60, 442, 1975.
10. Van Duuren, B. L. and Sivak, A., Tumor promoting agents from *Croton tiglium L.,* and their mode of action, *Cancer Res.,* 28, 2349, 1968.
11. Fujiki, H., Mori, M., Nakayasu, M., Sugimura, T., and Moore, R. E., Indole alkaloids: dihydroteleocidin B, teleocidin and lyngbytoxin A as members of a new class of tumor promoters, *Proc. Natl. Acad. Sci. U.S.A.,* 78, 3872, 1981.
12. Fujiki, H., Mori, M., Nakayasu, M., Terada, M., and Sugimura, T., A possible naturally occurring tumor promoter, teleocidin B, from *Streptomyces, Biochem. Biophys. Res. Commun.,* 90, 976, 1979.
13. Fujiki, H., Suganuma, M., Nakayasu, M., Hoshino, H., Moore, R. E., and Sugimura, T., A third class of new tumor promoters, polyacetates (debromoaplysiatoxin and aplysiatoxin) can differentiate biological actions relevant to tumor promoters, *Gann,* 73, 495, 1982.
14. Sugimura, T., Potent tumor promoters other than phorbol ester and their significance, *Gann,* 73, 499, 1982.
15. Laskin, J. D., Mufson, A., Piccinini, L., Engelhardt, D. L., and Weinstein, I. B., Effects of the tumor promoter 12-o-tetradecanoyl-phorbol-13-acetate on newly-synthesized proteins in mouse epidermis, *Cell,* 25, 441, 1981.
16. Viaje, A., Slaga, T. J., Wigler, M., and Weinstein, I. B., Effects of anti-inflammatory agents on mouse skin tumor promotion, epidermal DNA synthesis, phorbol ester-induced cellular proliferation, and production of plasminogen activator, *Cancer Res.,* 37, 1530, 1977.
17. Yuspa, S. H., Ben, T., and Hennings, H., The induction of epidermal transglutaminase and terminal differentiation by tumor promoters in cultured mouse epidermal cells, *Carcinogenesis,* 4, 1413, 1983.
18. O'Brien, T. G., Simisiman, R. C., and Boutwell, R. K., Induction of the polyamine biosynthetic enzymes in mouse epidermis by tumor promoting agents, *Cancer Res.,* 35, 1662, 1975.
19. Levine, L. and Hassid, A., Effects of phorbol-12,13-diesters on prostaglandin production and phospholipase activity in canine kidney (MDCK) cells, *Biochem. Biophys. Res. Commun.,* 79, 477, 1977.
20. Mufson, R. A., DeFeo, D., and Weinstein, I. B., Effect of phorbol ester tumor promoters on arachidonic acid metabolism in chick embryo fibroblasts, *Mol. Pharmacol.,* 16, 569, 1979.
21. Watanabe, T., Taguchi, Y., Kitamura, Y., Tsuyama, K., Fujiki, H., Tanooka, H., and Sugimura, T., Induction of histidine decarboxylase activity in mouse skin after application of indole alkaloids, a new class of tumor promoter, *Biochem. Biophys. Res. Commun.,* 109, 478, 1982.
22. Taguchi, Y., Tsuyama, K., Watanabe, T., Wada, H., and Kitamura, Y., Increase in histidine decarboxylase activity in skin of genetically mast-cell-deficient W/Wv mice after application of phorbol 12-myristate 13-acetate: evidence for the presence of histamine-producing cells without basophilic granules, *Proc. Natl. Acad. Sci. U.S.A.,* 79, 6837, 1982.
24. Mufson, R. A., Simisiman, R. C., and Boutwell, R. K., Increased cyclic adenosine 3':5'-monophosphate phosphodiesterase activity in the epidermis of phorbol ester-treated mouse skin and in papillomas, *Cancer Res.,* 39, 2036, 1979.

25. De Young, L. M., Argyris, R. S., and Gordon, G. B., Epidermal ribosome accumulation during two stage skin tumorigenesis, *Cancer Res.*, 37, 388, 1977.

26. Raineri, R., Simisiman, R. C., and Boutwell, R. K., Stimulation of the phosphorylation of mouse epidermal histones by tumor promoting agents, *Cancer Res.*, 33, 134, 1973.

27. O'Brien, T. G., The induction of ornithine decarboxylase as an early, possibly obligatory, event in mouse skin carcinogenesis, *Cancer Res.*, 36, 2644, 1976.

28. O'Brien, T. G., Lewis, M. A., and Diamond, L., Ornithine decarboxylase activity and DNA synthesis after treatment of cells in culture with 12-o-tetradecanoylphorbol-13-acetate, *Cancer Res.*, 39, 4477, 1979.

29. Yuspa, S. H., Lichti, U., Ben, T., Patterson, E., Hennings, H., Slaga, T. J., Colburn, N., and Kelsey, W., Phorbol esters stimulate DNA synthesis and ornithine decarboxylase activity in mouse epidermal cell cultures, *Nature (London)*, 262, 402, 1976.

30. Lesiewicz, J., Morrison, D. M., and Goldsmith, L. A., Ornithine decarboxylase in rat skin. II. Differential response to hairplucking and a tumor promoter, *J. Invest. Dermatol.*, 75, 411, 1980.

31. Bisschop, A., van Rooijen, L. A., Derks, H. J., and van Wijk, R., Induction of rat hepatic ornithine decarboxylase by the tumor promoters 12-o-tetradecanoylphorbol-13-acetate and phenobarbital *in vivo:* effect of retinyl-acetate, *Carcinogenesis*, 2, 1283, 1981.

32. Rifkin, D. B., Crowe, R. M., and Pollack, R., Tumor promoters induce changes in the chick embryo fibroblast cytoskeleton, *Cell*, 18, 361, 1979.

33. Ojakian, G. K., Tumor promoter-induced changes in the permeability of epithelial cell tight junctions, *Cell*, 23, 95, 1981.

34. Fisher, P. B., Young, C. S. H., Weinstein, I. B., and Carter, T. H., Tumor promoters alter the temporal program of adenovirus replication in human cells, *Mol. Cell. Biol.*, 1, 170, 1981.

35. Carter, T. H., Milovanovic, Z. Z., Babiss, L. E., and Fisher, P. B., Accelerated onset of viral transcription in adenovirus-infected HeLa cells treated with the tumor promoter 12-o-tetradecanoyl-phorbol-13-acetate, *Mol. Cell. Biol.*, 4, 563, 1984.

36. Kennedy, A., Promotion and other interactions between agents in the induction of transformation in vitro in fibroblasts, in *Mechanisms of Tumor Promotion: Tumor Promotion and Cocarcinogenesis In Vitro*, Slaga, J., Ed., CRC Press, Boca Raton, Fla., 1983, 14.

37. Slaga, T. J., Sivak, A., and Boutwell, R. K., Eds., *Carcinogenesis, Mechanisms of Tumor Promotion and Co-Carcinogenesis*, Raven Press, New York, 1978.

38. Brinckerhoff, C. E., Gross, R. H., Nagase, H., Sheldon, L., Jackson, R. C., and Harris, E. D., Jr., Increased level of translatable collagenase messenger ribonucleic acid in rabbit synovial fibroblasts treated with phorbol myristate acetate or crystals of monosodium urate monohydrate, *Biochemistry*, 21, 2674, 1982.

39. Hiwasa, T., Fujimura, S., and Sakiyama, S., Tumor promoters increase the synthesis of a 32,000-dalton protein in Balb/c 3T3 cells, *Proc. Natl. Acad. Sci. U.S.A.*, 79, 1800, 1982.

40. Yuspa, S. H., Lichti, U., Morgan, D., and Hennings, H., Chemical carcinogenesis studies in mouse epidermal cell cultures, *Curr. Probl. Dermatol.*, 10, 171, 1980.

41. Gottesman, M. M. and Sobel, M. E., Tumor promoters and Kirsten sarcoma virus increase synthesis of a secreted glycoprotein by regulating levels of a translatable mRNA, *Cell*, 19, 449, 1980.

42. Lichti, U. and Gottesman, M. M., Genetic evidence that a phorbol ester tumor promoter stimulates ornithine decarboxylase activity by a pathway that is independent of cyclic AMP-dependent protein kinases in CHO cells, *J. Cell. Physiol.*, 113, 433, 1982.

43. Fisher, P. B., Babiss, L. E., Weinstein, I. B., and Ginsberg, H. S., Analysis of type 5 adenovirus transformation with a cloned rat embryo cell line (CREF), *Proc. Natl. Acad. Sci. U.S.A.*, 79, 3527, 1982.

44. Fisher, P. B., Enhancement of viral transformation and expression of the transformed phenotype by tumor promoters, in *Mechanisms of Tumor Promotion: Tumor Promotion and Cocarcinogenesis In Vitro*, Slaga, J., Ed., CRC Press, Boca Raton, Fla., 1983, 57.

45. Vandenbark, G. R. and Niedel, J. E., Phorbol esters and cellular differentiation, *J. Natl. Cancer Inst.*, 73, 1013, 1984.

46. Lasne, C., Gentil, A., and Chouroulinkov, I., Two stage malignant transformation of rat fibroblasts in tissue culture, *Nature (London)*, 247, 490, 1974.

47. Mondal, S., Brankow, D. W., and Heidelberger, C., Two-stage chemical oncogenesis in cultures of C3H/10T₁□₂ cells, *Cancer Res.*, 36, 2254, 1976.

48. Mondal, S. and Heidelberger, C., Transformation of C3H/10T₁□₂ Cl 8 mouse embryo fibroblasts by ultraviolet radiation and a phorbol ester, *Nature (London)*, 260, 710, 1976.

49. Kennedy, A., Mondal, S., Heidelberger, C., and Little, J. B., Enhancement of X-irradiation transformation by 12-o-tetradecanoyl-phorbol-13-acetate in a cloned line of C3H mouse embryo cells, *Cancer Res.*, 38, 439, 1978.

50. Fisher, P. B., Mufson, R. A., Weinstein, I. B., and Little, J. B., Epidermal growth factor, like tumor promoters, enhances viral and radiation-induced cell transformation, *Carcinogenesis,* 2, 183, 1981.

51. Fisher, P. B., Weinstein, I. B., Eisenberg, D., and Ginsberg, H. S., Interactions between adenovirus, a tumor promoter and chemical carcinogens in the transformation of rat embryo cells in culture, *Proc. Natl. Acad. Sci. U.S.A.,* 75, 2311, 1978.

52. Martin, R. G., Setlow, V. P., Edwards, C. A. F., and Vembu, D., The role of simian virus 40 tumor antigens in transformation of Chinese hamster lung cells, *Cell,* 17, 636, 1979.

53. Monier, R., Cell transformation by simian virus 40 mutants, *Int. Symp. Princess Takamatsu Cancer Res. Fund,* 12, 263, 1982.

54. Seif, R., Factors which disorganize microfilaments increase the frequency of transformation by polyoma virus, *J. Virol.,* 36, 421, 1980.

55. Yamamoto, N. and zur Hausen, H., Tumor promoter TPA enhances transformation of human leukocytes by Epstein-Barr virus, *Nature (London),* 280, 244, 1979.

56. Amtmann, E. and Sauer, G., Activation of non-expressed bovine papilloma genomes by tumor promoters, *Nature (London),* 296, 675, 1982.

57. O'Brien, T. G. and Diamond, L., Ornithine decarboxylase induction and DNA synthesis in hamster embryo cell cultures treated with tumor-promoting phorbol diesters, *Cancer Res.,* 37, 3895, 1977.

58. O'Brien, T. G., Daladik, D., and Diamond, L., Regulation of polyamine biosynthesis in normal and transformed hamster cells in culture, *Biochim. Biophys. Acta,* 632, 270, 1980.

59. Guy, G. R. and Murray, A. W., Modulation of HeLa cell phospholipid metabolism and ornithine-decarboxylase activity by tumor promoters: regulation of response to phorbol-12,13-dibutyrate by receptor occupancy time, *Biochem. Biophys. Res. Commun.,* 106, 1398, 1982.

60. Wu, V. S. and Byus, C. V., The induction of ornithine decarboxylase by tumor promoting phorbol ester analogs in Reuber H35 hepatoma cells, *Life Sci.,* 29, 1855, 1981.

61. Paranjpe, M. S., De Larco, J. E., and Todaro, G. J., Retinoids block ornithine decarboxylase induction in cells treated with the tumor promoter TPA or the peptide growth hormones, EGF and SGF, *Biochem. Biophys. Res. Commun.,* 94, 586, 1980.

62. Dion, L. D., Bear, J., Bateman, J., DeLuca, L. M., and Colburn, N. H., Tumor promoting phorbol ester inhibits procollagen synthesis in promotable JB-6 mouse epidermal cells, *J. Natl. Cancer Inst.,* 69, 1147, 1982.

63. Dion, L. D., De Luca, L. M., and Colburn, N. H., Phorbol ester-induced anchorage independence and its antagonism by retinoic acid correlates with altered expression of specific glycoproteins, *Carcinogenesis,* 2, 951, 1981.

64. Sobel, M. E., Dion, L. D., Vuust, J., and Colburn, N. H., Tumor-promoting phorbol esters inhibit procollagen synthesis at a pretranslational level in JB-6 mouse cells, *Mol. Cell. Biol.,* 3, 1527, 1983.

65. Hiawasa, T., Fujiki, H., Sugimura, T., and Sakiyama, S., Increase in the synthesis of a Mr 32,000 protein in Balb/c 3T3 cells treated with tumor-promoting indole alkaloids or polyacetates, *Cancer Res.,* 42, 5951, 1983.

66. Gottesman, M. M. and Cabral, F., Purification and characterization of a transformation-dependent protein secreted by cultured murine fibroblasts, *Biochemistry,* 20, 1659, 1981.

67. Gottesman, M. M., Transformation-dependent secretion of a low molecular weight protein by murine fibroblasts, *Proc. Natl. Acad. Sci. U.S.A.,* 75, 2767, 1978.

68. Hennings, H., Michal, D., Cheng, C., Steinert, P., Holbrook, K., and Yuspa, S. H., Calcium regulation of growth and differentiation of mouse epidermal cells in culture, *Cell,* 19, 245, 1980.

69. Tarone, G., Ceschi, P., Prat, M., and Comoglio, P. M., Transformation sensitive protein with molecular weight of 45,000 secreted by mouse fibroblasts, *Cancer Res.,* 41, 3648, 1981.

70. Cabral, F., Gottesman, M. M., and Yuspa, S. H., Induction of specific protein synthesis by phorbol esters in mouse epidermal cell culture, *Cancer Res.,* 41, 2025, 1981.

71. Yuspa, S. H., Ben, T., Hennings, H., and Lichti, U., Divergent responses in basal epidermal cells to the tumor promoter 12-o-tetradecanoylphorbol-13-acetate, *Cancer Res.,* 42, 2344, 1982.

72. Yuspa, S. H., Ben, T., and Lichti, U., Regulation of epidermal transglutaminase activity and terminal differentiation by retinoids and phorbol esters, *Cancer Res.,* 83, 5707, 1983.

73. Yuspa, S. H., Ben, T., Hennings, H., and Lichti, U., Phorbol ester tumor promoters induce epidermal transglutaminase activity, *Biochem. Biophys. Res. Commun.,* 97, 700, 1980.

74. Yuspa, S. H., Lichti, U., Morgan, D., and Hennings, H., Chemical carcinogenesis studies in mouse epidermal cell culture, in *Biochemistry of Normal and Abnormal Epidermal Differentiation,* Bernstein, I. A. and Seiji, M., Eds., University of Tokyo Press, Tokyo, 1980, 171.

75. Kawamura, H., Strickland, J. E., and Yuspa, S. H., Inhibition of 12-o-tetradecanoylphorbol-13-acetate induction of epidermal transglutaminase activity by protease inhibitors, *Cancer Res.,* 43, 4073, 1983.

76. Verma, A. K., Froscio, M., and Murray, A. W., Croton oil and benzo(a)pyrene-induced changes in cyclic adenosine 3′:5′-monophosphate and cyclic guanosine 3′:5′-monophosphate phosphodiesterase activities in mouse epidermis, *Cancer Res.*, 36, 81, 1976.

76a. West, C. V. M. and Holtzer, H., Protein synthesis and degradation in cultured muscle is altered by a phorbol diester tumor promoter, *Arch. Biochem. Biophys.*, 219, 335, 1982.

77. Cossu, G., Pasifici, M., Adamo, S., Bouche, M., and Molinaro, M., TPA-inhibition of the expression of differentiative traits in cultured myotubes: dependence on protein synthesis, *Differentiation*, 21, 62, 1982.

78. Brinckerhoff, C. E. and Harris, E. D., Jr., Modulation by retinoic acid and corticosteroids of collagenase production by rabbit synovial fibroblasts treated with phorbolmyristate acetate or poly(ethylene glycol), *Biochim. Biophys. Acta*, 677, 424, 1981.

79. Aggeler, J., Frisch, S., and Werb, Z., Collagenase is a major gene product of induced rabbit synovial fibroblasts, *J. Cell Biol.*, 98, 1656, 1984.

80. Aggeler, J., Firsch, S. M., and Werb, Z., Changes in cell shape correlate with collagenase gene expression in rabbit synovial fibroblasts, *J. Cell Biol.*, 98, 1662, 1984.

81. Laszlo, A., Radke, K., Chin, S., and Bissell, M. J., Tumor promoters alter gene expression and protein phosphorylation in avian cells in culture, *Proc. Natl. Acad. Sci. U.S.A.*, 78, 6241, 1981.

82. Chida, K. and Kuroki, T., Inhibition of DNA synthesis and sugar uptake and lack of induction of ornithine decarboxylase in human epidermal cells treated with mouse skin tumor promoters, *Cancer Res.*, 44, 875, 1984.

83. Schopp, M., Mellick, U., Rahmsdorf, H. J., and Herrlich, P., UV-induced extracellular factor from human fibroblasts communicates the UV response to nonirradiated cells, *Cell*, 37, 861, 1984.

84. Soprano, K. J. and Baserga, R., Reactivation of ribosomal genes in human-mouse hybrid cells by 12-o-tetradecanoyl-phorbol-13-acetate, *Proc. Natl. Acad. Sci. U.S.A.*, 77, 1566, 1980.

85. Bleackley, R. C., Caplan, B., Havele, C., Rtizel, R. G., Mosman, T. R., Farrar, J. J., and Paetkau, V., Translation of lymphocyte mRNA into biologically-active interleukin 2 in oocytes, *J. Immunol.*, 127, 2432, 1981.

86. Hoffman-Liebermann, B., Liebermann, D., and Sachs, L., Regulation of gene expression by tumor promoters. III. Complementation of the developmental program in myeloid leukemic cells by regulating mRNA production and mRNA translation, *Int. J. Cancer*, 28, 615, 1981.

87. Liebermann, D., Hoffman-Liebermann, B., and Sachs, L., Regulation of gene expression by tumor promoters. II. Control of cell shape and developmental programs for macrophages and granulocytes in human myeloid leukemia cells, *Int. J. Cancer*, 28, 285, 1981.

88. Sachs, L., Constitutive uncoupling of pathways of gene expression that control growth and differentiation in myeloid leukemia: a model for the origin and progression of malignancy, *Proc. Natl. Acad. Sci. U.S.A.*, 77, 6152, 1980.

89. Crutchley, D. J., Conan, L. B., and Maynard, J. R., Induction of plasminogen activator and prostaglandin biosynthesis in HeLa cells by 12-o-tetradecanoylphorbol-13-acetate, *Cancer Res.*, 40, 849, 1980.

90. Guy, K., Van Heyningen, V., Dewar, E., and Steele, C. M., Enhanced expression of human Ia antigens by chronic lymphocytic leukemia cells following treatment with 12-o-tetradecanoylphorbol-13-acetate, *Eur. J. Immunol.*, 13, 156, 1983.

91. Ashino-Fuse, H., Opdenaker, G., Fuse, A., and Billiau, A., Mechanism of the stimulatory effect of phorbol 12-myristate 13 acetate on cellular production of plasminogen activator, *Proc. Soc. Exp. Biol. Med.*, 176, 109, 1984.

92. de Bustros, A., Baylin, S. B., Berger, C. L., Roos, B. A., Leong, S. S., and Belkin, B., Phorbol esters increase calcitonin gene transcription and decrease c-myc levels in cultured human medullary thyroid carcinoma, *J. Biol. Chem.*, 260, 98, 1985.

93. Campisi, J., Gray, H. E., Pardee, A. B., Dean, M., and Sonenshein, G. E., Cell cycle control of c-myc but not c-ras expression is lost following chemical transformation, *Cell*, 36, 241, 1984.

94. Kelley, K., Cochran, B. H., Stiles, C. D., and Leder, P., Cell-specific regulation of the c-myc gene by lymphocyte mitogens and platelet-derived growth factor, *Cell*, 35, 603, 1983.

95. Craig, R. W. and Bloch, A., Early decline in c-myb oncogene expression in the differentiation of human myeloblastic leukemia (ML-1) cells induced with 12-o-tetradecanoyl-phorbol-13-acetate, *Cancer Res.*, 44, 442, 1984.

96. Greenberg, M. E. and Ziff, E. B., Stimulation of 3T3 cells induces transcription of the c-fos proto-oncogene, *Nature (London)*, 311, 433, 1984.

97. Muller, R., Bravo, R., and Burckhardt, J., Induction of c-fos gene and protein by growth factors precedes activation of c-myc, *Nature (London)*, 312, 716, 1984.

98. Kruijer, W., Cooper, J. A., Hunter, T., and Verma, I. M., Platelet-derived growth factor induces rapid but transient expression of the c-fos gene and protein, *Nature (London)*, 312, 711, 1984.

99. Cochran, B. H., Zullo, J., Verma, I. M., and Stiles, C. D., Expression of the c-fos gene and of an fos-related gene is stimulated by platelet-derived growth factor, *Science,* 226, 1080, 1984.

100. Murdoch, G. H., Evans, R. M., and Rosenfeld, M. G., Polypeptide hormone regulation of gene expression. Thyrotropin-releasing hormone rapidly stimulates both transcription of the prolactin gene and the phosphorylation of a specific nuclear protein, *J. Biol. Chem.,* 258, 15329, 1983.

101. Granner, D., Andreone, T., Kazuyuki, S., and Beale, E., Inhibition of transcription of the phosphoenolpyruvate carboxykinase gene by insulin, *Nature (London),* 305, 549, 1983.

102. Schonbrunn, A., Krasnoff, M., Westendorf, J. M., and Tashjian, A. H., Jr., Epidermal growth factor and thyrotropin-releasing hormone act similarly on a clonal pituitary cell strain, *J. Cell Biol.,* 85, 786, 1980.

103. Johnson, L. K., Baxter, J. D., Vladavsky, I., and Gospodarowicz, D., Epidermal growth factor and expression of specific genes: effects on cultured rat pituitary cells are dissociable from the mitogenic response, *Proc. Natl. Acad. Sci. U.S.A.,* 77, 394, 1980.

104. Osborne, R. and Tasjian, A. J., Jr., Tumor promoting phorbol esters affect production of prolactin and growth hormone by pituitary cells, *Endocrinology,* 108, 1164, 1981.

105. Supowit, S. C., Potter, E., Evans, R. M., and Rosenfeld, M. G., Polypeptide regulation of gene transcription: specific 5′ genomic sequences are required for epidermal growth factor and phorbol ester regulation of prolactin gene expression, *Proc. Natl. Acad. Sci. U.S.A.,* 81, 2975, 1984.

106. Cooke, N. E. and Baxter, J. D., Structural analysis of the prolactin gene suggests a separate origin for its 5′ end, *Nature (London),* 297, 603, 1982.

107. Pietropaolo, C., Laskin, J. A., and Weinstein, I. B., Effect of tumor promoters on sarc gene expression in normal and transformed chick embryo fibroblasts, *Cancer Res.,* 41, 1565, 1981.

108. Finkel, M. P., Biskis, B. O., and Jinkins, P. B., Virus induction of osteosarcomas in mice, *Science,* 151, 698, 1966.

109. Curran, T., Miller, A. D., Zokas, L., and Verma, I. M., Viral and cellular fos proteins: a comparative analysis, *Cell,* 36, 259, 1984.

110. Van Breveren, C., van Straaten, F., Curran, T., Muller, R., and Verma, I. M., Analysis of FBJ-MuSV provirus and c-fos (mouse) gene reveals that viral and cellular fos gene products have different carboxy termini, *Cell,* 32, 1241, 1983.

111. van Straaten, F., Curran, T., Van Breveren, C., and Verma, I. M., Complete nucleotide sequence of a human onc gene: deduced amino acid sequence of the human c-fos protein, *Proc. Natl. Acad. Sci. U.S.A.,* 80, 3183, 1983.

112. Muller, R. and Verma, I. M., Expression of cellular oncogenes, *Curr. Top. Microbiol. Immunol.,* 112, 73, 1984.

113. Mitchell, R. L., Zokas, L., Schreiber, R. D., and Verma, I. M., Rapid induction of the expression of proto-oncogene fos during human monocytic differentiation, *Cell,* 40, 209, 1985.

114. Miller, A. D., Curran, T., and Verma, I. M., C-fos protein can induce cellular transformation: a novel mechanism of activation of a cellular oncogene, *Cell,* 36, 51, 1984.

115. Berk, A. J., Lee, F., Harrison, T., Williams, J., and Sharp, P. A., Pre-early adenovirus 5 gene product regulates synthesis of early viral messenger RNAs, *Cell,* 17, 935, 1979.

116. Weeks, D. L. and Jones, N. C., Ela control of gene expression is mediated by sequences 5′ to the transcriptional starts of early viral genes, *Mol. Cell. Biol.,* 3, 1222, 1983.

117. Nevins, J. R., Mechanism of activation of early virus transcription by the adenovirus Ela gene product, *Cell,* 26, 213, 1981.

118. Nevins, J. R., Ginsberg, H. S., Blanchard, J.-M., Wilson, M. C., and Darnell, J. E., Regulation of the primary expression of the early adenovirus transcription units, *J. Virol.,* 32, 727, 1979.

119. Weinberg, R. A., Cellular oncogenes, *Trends Biochem. Sci.,* April, 131, 1984.

120. Katze, M. G., Persson, H., Johansson, B. M., and Philipson, L., Control of adenovirus gene expression: cellular gene products restrict expression of adenovirus host range mutants in nonpermissive cells, *J. Virol.,* 46, 50, 1983.

121. Arya, S. K., Phorbol ester-mediated stimulation of the synthesis of mouse mammary tumor virus, *Nature (London),* 284, 71, 1980.

122. Kwon, B. S. and Weissman, S. M., Mouse mammary tumor virus-related sequences in mouse lymphocytes are inducible by 12-o-tetradecanoyl phorbol-13-acetate, *J. Virol.,* 52, 1000, 1984.

123. zur Hausen, H., Oncogenic herpes viruses, *Biochim. Biophys. Acta,* 417, 25, 1975.

124. Hinuma, Y., Konn, M., Yamaguchi, J., Wudarski, D. J., Blakeslee, J. R., and Grace, J. T., Immunofluorescence and herpes-type virus particles in the P3HR-1 Burkitt lymphoma cell line, *J. Virol.,* 1, 1045, 1967.

125. Gerber, P., Activation of Epstein-Barr virus by 5-bromo-deoxyuridine in virus free human cells, *Proc. Natl. Acad. Sci. U.S.A.,* 69, 83, 1972.

126. Bister, K., Yamamoto, N., and zur Hausen, H., Differential inducibility of Epstein-Barr virus in cloned, non-producer Raji cells, *Int. J. Cancer,* 23, 818, 1979.

127. Klein, G. and Dambos, L., Relationship between the sensitivity of EBV-carrying lymphoblastoid lines to superinfection and the inducibility of the residential viral genome, *Int. J. Cancer,* 11, 327, 1973.

128. zur Hausen, H., Bornkamm, G. W., Schmidt, R., and Hecker, E., Tumor initiators and promoters in the induction of Epstein-Barr virus, *Proc. Natl. Acad. Sci. U.S.A.,* 76, 782, 1979.

129. zur Hausen, H., O'Niell, F. J., and Freeze, J. K., Persisting oncogenic herpes virus induced by the promoter TPA, *Nature (London),* 272, 373, 1978.

130. Shin, S., Donovan, J., and Nonoyama, M., Phosphonoacetic acid-resistant RNA of Epstein-Barr virus in productively infected cells, *Virology,* 124, 196, 1983.

131. Shin, S., Tanaka, A., and Nonoyama, M., Transcription of the Epstein-Barr virus genome in productively infected cells, *Virology,* 124, 13, 1983.

132. Jeang, K. T. and Hayward, S. D., Organization of the Epstein-Barr virus DNA molecule. III. Location of the P3HR-1 deletion junction and characterization of the Not1 repeat units that form part of the template for an abundant 12-o-tetradecanoyl-phorbol-13-acetate-induced mRNA transcript, *J. Virol.,* 48, 135, 1983.

133. Biggin, M., Farrell, P. J., and Barrell, B. G., Transcription and DNA sequence of the BamHI L fragment of B95-8 Epstein-Barr virus, *EMBO J.,* 3, 1083, 1984.

134. Allaudeen, H. S. and Rani, G., Cellular and Epstein-Barr virus specific DNA polymerase in virus-producing Burkitt's lymphoma cell lines, *Nucleic Acids Res.,* 10, 2453, 1982.

135. Weigel, R. and Miller, G., Major EB virus-specific cytoplasmic transcripts in a cellular clone of the HR-1 Burkitt lymphoma line during latency and after induction of the viral replicative cycle by phorbol esters, *Virology,* 125, 287, 1983.

136. Lin, J. C., Smith, M. C., and Pagano, J. S., Activation of latent Epstein-Barr virus genomes: selective stimulation of synthesis of chromosomal proteins by a tumor promoter, *J. Virol.,* 45, 985, 1983.

137. Krieg, P., Amtman, E., and Sauer, G., Interaction between latent papovavirus genomes and the tumor promoter TPA, *FEBS Lett.,* 128, 191, 1981.

138. Goldberg, A. R., Delclos, K. B., and Blumberg, P. M., Phorbol ester action is independent of viral and cellular src kinase levels, *Science,* 208, 191, 1980.

139. lipp, M., Scherer, B., Lips, G., Brandner, G., and Hunsman, G., Diverse effects: augmentation, inhibition and non-efficacy of 12-o-tetradecanoyl-phorbol-13-acetate (TPA) on retrovirus genome expression in vitro and in vivo, *Carcinogenesis,* 3, 261, 1982.

140. Hellman, K. B. and Helman, A., Induction of type-C retroviruses by the tumor promoter TPA, *Int. J. Cancer,* 27, 95, 1981.

141. Hoshino, H., Miwa, M., and Fujiki, H., A new tumor promoter, dihydroteleocidin B, enhances cell growth and the production of murine leukemia virus by fibroblasts, *Int. J. Cancer,* 31, 509, 1983.

142. Wunderlich, V., Baumbach, L., and Sydow, G., Tumor promoter-stimulated synthesis of Mason-Pfizer monkey virus, *Cancer Res. Clin. Oncol.,* 102, 271, 1982.

143. Weinstein, I. B., Lee, L. S., Fisher, P. B., Mufson, A., and Yamasaki, H., Cellular and biochemical events associated with the action of tumor promoters, in *Naturally Occurring Carcinogens, Mutagens and Modulators of Carcinogenesis,* Miller, E. C. et al., Eds., University Park Press, Baltimore, 1979, 301.

144. Weinstein, I. B., Wigler, M., Fisher, P. B., Sisskin, E., and Pietropaolo, C., Cell culture studies on the biologic effects of tumor promoters, in *Carcinogenesis, Mechanisms of Tumor Promotion and Cocarcinogenesis,* Vol. 2, Slaga, T. J., Sivak, A., and Boutwell, R. K., Eds., Raven Press, New York, 1978, 313.

145. Carpenter, G. and Cohan, S., Peptide growth factors, *Trends in Biochem. Sci.,* April, 169, 1984.

146. Nishizuka, Y., Protein kinases in signal transduction, *Trends in Biochem. Sci.,* April, 163, 1984.

147. Blumberg, P. M., Jaken, S., Konig, B., Sharkey, N. A., Leach, K. L., Yeng, A. Y., and Yeh, E., Mechanism of action of phorbol ester tumor promoters: specific receptors for lipophilic ligands, *Biochem. Pharmacol.,* 33, 933, 1984.

148. Friedman, B., Frackelton, A. R., Jr., Ross, A. H., Connors, J. M., Fujiki, H., Sugimura, T., and Rosner, M. R., Tumor promoters block tyrosine-specific phosphorylation of the epidermal growth factor, *Proc. Natl. Acad. Sci. U.S.A.,* 81, 3034, 1984.

149. Hunter, T., The epidermal growth factor receptor gene and its product, *Nature (London),* 311, 414, 1984.

150. Belman, S. and Troll, W., The inhibition of croton oil promoted mouse skin tumorigenesis by steroid hormones, *Cancer Res.,* 32, 450, 1972.

151. Slaga, T. J., Antiinflammatory steroids: potent inhibitors of tumor promotion, in *Carcinogenesis,* Vol. 5, *Modifiers of Chemical Carcinogenesis,* Slaga, T. J., Ed., Raven Press, New York, 1980, 111.

152. Sundar, S. K., Ablashi, D. V., Armstrong, G. R., Zipkin, M., Faggioni, A., and Levine, P. H., Steroids inhibit tumor promoting agent induced Epstein-Barr virus early antigens in Raji cells, *Int. J. Cancer,* 28, 503, 1981.

153. Schmidt, N. J., Improved yields and assay of simian varicella virus, and a comparison of certain biological properties of simian and human varicella viruses, *J. Virol. Methodol.*, 5, 229, 1982.
154. Logan, J. S. and Shenk, T., Transcriptional and translational control of adenovirus gene expression, *Microbiol. Rev.*, 46, 377, 1982.
155. Blanton, R. A. and Carter, T. H., Autoregulation of adenovirus type 5 gene expression. III. Transcription studies in isolated nuclei, *J. Virol.*, 29, 458, 1979.
156. Carter, T. H. and Blanton, R. A., Possible role of the 72,000 dalton DNA-binding protein in regulation of adenovirus type 5 early gene expression, *J. Virol.*, 25, 664, 1978.
157. Nevins, J. R. and Jensen-Winkler, J. J., Regulation of early adenovirus transcription: a protein product of early region 2 specifically represses region 4 transcription, *Proc. Natl. Acad. Sci. U.S.A.*, 77, 1893, 1980.
158. Babich, A. and Nevins, J. R., The stability of early adenovirus mRNA is controlled by the viral 72 kd DNA-binding protein, *Cell*, 26, 371, 1981.
159. Katze, M. G., Persson, H., and Philipson, L., Control of adenovirus gene expression: post transcriptional control mediated by both viral and cellular gene products, *Mol. Cell. Biol.*, 1, 807, 1981.
160. Ricciardi, R. P., Jones, R. L., Cepko, C. L., Sharp, P. A., and Roberts, B. E., Expression of early adenovirus genes requires a viral encoded acidic polypeptide, *Proc. Natl. Acad. Sci. U.S.A.*, 78, 6121, 1981.
161. Van Ormondt, H., Maat, J., de Waard, A., and van der Eb, A. J., The nucleotide sequence of the transforming early region of adenovirus type 5 DNA, *Gene*, 11, 299, 1980.
162. Gaynor, R. B. and Berk, A. J., Cis-acting induction of adenovirus transcription, *Cell*, 33, 683, 1983.
163. Feldman, L. T. and Nevins, J. R., Localization of the adenovirus Ela protein, a positive-acting transcriptional factor, in infected cells, *Mol. Cell. Biol.*, 3, 829, 1983.
164. Zakeri-Milovanovic, Z., Mechanism of Enhancement of Type 5 Adenovirus Early Gene Expression by the Tumor Promoter 12-o-Tetradecanoyl-Phorbol-13-Acetate, Ph.D. thesis, St. John's University, Jamaica, New York, 1984.
165. Wessels, N. K., Spooner, B. S., and Ash, J. F., Microfilaments in cellular and developmental processes, *Science*, 171, 135, 1971.
166. Schiff, P. B., Fant, J., and Horowitz, S. B., Promotion of microtubule assembly in vitro by taxol, *Nature (London)*, 277, 665, 1979.
167. Olmsted, J. B. and Borisy, G. C., Microtubules, *Annu. Rev. Biochem.*, 42, 507, 1973.
168. Babiss, L. E., Fisher, P. B., and Ginsberg, H. S., Deletion and insertion mutations in early region 1a of type 5 adenovirus that produce cold-sensitive or defective phenotypes for transformation, *J. Virol.*, 49, 731, 1984.
169. Weinmann, R., Brandler, T. G., Raskas, H. J., and Roeder, R. G., Low molecular weight RNAs transcribed by RNA polymerase III during adenovirus 2 infection, *Cell*, 7, 557, 1976.
170. Weinmann, R., Jaening, J. A., Raskas, H. J., and Roeder, R. G., Viral RNA synthesis and levels of DNA-dependent RNA polymerases during replication of adenovirus 2, *J. Virol.*, 17, 114, 1976.
171. Manley, J. A., Sharp, P. A., and Gefter, M. L., RNA synthesis in isolated nuclei: identification and comparison of adenovirus 2 encoded transcripts synthesized in vitro and in vivo, *J. Mol. Biol.*, 135, 171, 1979.
172. Manley, J. L., Sharp, P. A., and Gefter, M. L., RNA synthesis in isolated nuclei: in vitro initiation of adenovirus 2 major late mRNA precursor, *Proc. Natl. Acad. Sci. U.S.A.*, 76, 160, 1979.
173. Fire, A. C., Baker, J., Manley, J., Ziff, E., and Sharp, P., In vitro transcription of adenovirus, *J. Virol.*, 40, 703, 1981.
174. Handa, H., Kaufman, R., Manley, J., Gefter, M., and Sharp, P. A., Transcription of simian virus 40 DNA in a HeLa whole cell extract, *J. Biol. Chem.*, 256, 478, 1981.
175. Manley, J., Fire, A., Cano, A., Sharp, P. A., and Gefter, M., DNA-dependent transcription of adenovirus genes in a soluble whole cell extract, *Proc. Natl. Acad. Sci. U.S.A.*, 77, 3855, 1980.
176. Manley, J. M., Accurate and specific polyadenylation of mRNA precursors in a soluble whole cell lysate, *Cell*, 33, 595, 1983.
177. Parrella, F. W., Takigawa, M., and Boutwell, R. K., Purification of 12-o-tetradecanoylphorbol-13-acetate-induced ornithine decarboxylase from mouse epidermis, *Int. J. Biochem.*, 15, 885, 1983.
178. Scribner, J. D. and Van Duuren, B. L., RNA synthesis induction in cell culture by a tumor promoter, *Cancer Res.*, 30, 1203, 1970.
179. Trewyn, R. W. and Gatz, H. B., Altered growth properties of normal human cells induced by phorbol-12,13-didecanoate, *In Vitro*, 20, 409, 1984.
180. zur Hausen, H., Yamamoto, N., and Bauer, G., Virus induction by tumor promoters, *Carcinogen. Compr. Surv.*, 7, 69, 1982.
181. Ziff, E., personal communication, 1985.
182. Sauer, G., personal communication.
183. Zareki, Z. and Carter, T. H., unpublished information.

genic response to TPA[41] and teleocidin,[42] another tumor promoter with high affinity binding to the phorbol ester receptor. The resistant variants were unaffected in their arachidonic acid and prostaglandin release[43] and glucose uptake responses,[44] but showed resistance to TPA-enhanced gene amplification.[45] Although the basis for the resistance to TPA-induced mitogenesis is still being sought, mitogenic stimulation appears to be required for enhancement of gene amplification by TPA.

Colburn et al.[46] have described variants of JB6 mouse epidermal cells that are resistant to mitogenic stimulation by TPA. These variants showed diminished glucose uptake response[47] and lack of EGF receptors.[12] That the latter may be required for mitogenic response to TPA in JB6 cells was suggested by the finding that reconstitution of the resistant variants with EGF receptors in the form of unpurified membranes, yielded a restoration of mitogenic response not only to EGF but also to TPA.[48] Mitogenic responsiveness to TPA is not necessarily correlated to, and in fact can be dissociated from, the sensitivity to promotion of neoplastic transformation in JB6 cells, as demonstrated by the occurrence of mitogenesis-resistant promotion sensitive variants.[46] Perhaps establishment in culture serves a function similar to chronic hyperplasiagenic stimulation in vivo. In any case, the mitogenesis independence of the transformation-promoting response in JB6 cells facilitates the search for promotion-relevant events by allowing one to separate some of the many responses to TPA onto a "mitogenesis-specific" or a "promotion-specific" pathway.

F. Differentiation Response Variants

TPA and congeners such as teleocidin induce differentiation in human HL-60 promyelocytic leukemia cells,[49] and inhibit induced differentiation in mouse Friend erythroleukemia cells.[17] Resistant variants of both cell lines have been reported[17,49-51] but the basis for resistance to the TPA-induced differentiation responses is not known. Another class of differentiation-resistant cells has been described by Hennings et al.[52] and Yuspa et al.[53,54] These are putatively initiated mouse keratinocyte cell lines which are resistant to induction of terminal differentiation by high calcium or by TPA. Although this resistance provides a clear basis for *selective* growth advantages, such variants may also be valuable in elucidating tumor-promoter *induced* promotion-relevant responses to TPA. Both tumorigenic human keratinocytes and a subpopulation of normal human keratinocytes have been reported to be resistant to TPA-induced terminal differentiation.[55] Human bronchial epithelial tumor cells show a similar resistance to TPA-induced terminal differentiation.[56]

G. Cytotoxicity Variants

Human cells from donors carrying certain cancer-prone genetic disorders, or from those harboring certain DNA tumor viral genes, show altered sensitivity to cytotoxic effects of TPA. Fibroblasts of ataxia telangectasia individuals showed elevated cytotoxicity responses to TPA.[57] Human lymphoma cells showed increased TPA resistance if they harbored Epstein Barr virus genomes.[58]

H. Variants for Promotion or Progression of Transformation

A case of what may be sensitive variants for transformation promotion has been described for fibroblasts from humans showing the FP coli trait.[6] In this case, sensitivity to TPA-induced progression to anchorage independence (as reported earlier),[59] but not to tumorigenicity, was demonstrated.[6] In another report,[60] neither FP fibroblasts nor those from certain other genetically cancer-prone individuals were found to be sensitive to TPA-induced anchorage independence.

Rodent cell variants for induction or progression of neoplastic transformation by tumor promoters have been described. In several instances, integrated DNA tumor virus genes or *onc* genes confer promotion (or progression) sensitivity. These include adenovirus-5 transformed (Ad5) rat embryo fibroblasts,[61,62] rat fibroblasts transfected with polyoma large T (pyLT) or *myc* genes[63] and $10T_{1/2}$ mouse fibroblasts transfected with T24 DNA containing activated *H-ras* gene.[64] Recent evidence[87] indicates that one can produce an initiated or promotion-sensitive state in mice by exposure of "scratched" skin to Harvey sarcoma virus, suggesting that promotion sensitivity in vivo may also be produced by expression of an activated *H-ras* oncogene. A similar event may produce the initiated state in the case of NMU (*N*-nitroso-methyl-urea)-initiated rat mammary carcinogenesis.[65] In this case, the "tumor-promotion" stage is presumably brought about by the action of certain hormones. In this instance, unlike that involving the mouse epidermal experiments described earlier, it is not clear whether activation of the *H-ras* oncogene, which does occur, produces sensitivity to hormone-mediated preneoplastic progression.

Promotion sensitivity was acquired spontaneously in the case of JB6 mouse epidermal cells.[21,66,67] The sensitive cells in both this case and that of the Ad5 rat fibroblasts are induced to undergo enhanced anchorage independence and other growth changes in response to tumor-promoting (but not nonpromoting) phorbol esters, teleocidin, and EGF. In both JB6 cells and Ad5 cells, the response is irreversible, at least with a high frequency. The Ad5 fibroblasts are, in contrast to the JB6 cells and the pyLT or *myc* transformed fibroblasts, tumorigenic at the outset.[68] TPA produces *progression* of the Ad5 cells to a phenotype showing a shorter latent period for tumor formation and higher colony yield in agar.[61,62,68] TPA produces *promotion* of PyLT or *myc*-transfected fibroblasts to a tumor cell phenotype characterized by focus formation and anchorage-independent colony formation. The TPA-induced response of T24 transfected $10T_{1/2}$ cells may also consist of promotion from a nontumor- to a tumor-cell phenotype; clarification of this awaits demonstration of the tumorigenicity status of the cells prior to TPA exposure.

The promotion-sensitive (P+) JB6 cell lines undergo anchorage-independent transformation in response to TPA that is 100-fold greater than that in the resistant variants. The induced anchorage-independent transformants (but not untreated P+ JB6 cells) are tumorigenic. The irreversibility of JB6 cell transformation to tumorigenic phenotype appears to parallel late-stage tumor promotion in mouse skin. In the latter case, the commitment to TPA-dependent carcinoma induction has been irreversibly achieved by the papilloma stage.[69] Dominance of the P+ phenotype (which also occurs in vivo in mouse skin)[2] was demonstrated by cell fusion experiments.[70] That genes specifying promotion sensitivity could be expected, was demonstrated by transfection of DNA from sensitive (P+) donors into insensitive (P-) recipient cells.[71]

III. GENES THAT CONFER SUSCEPTIBILITY TO PROMOTION OF TRANSFORMATION (*pro*) GENES

A. Cloning and Characterization of *pro* Genes

As indicated earlier, several lines of evidence have suggested that a specific gene (or genes) might determine specific events in tumor promotion. Recently, Lerman et al.[72] have described the molecular cloning of two new genes that appear to confer susceptibility to promotion of neoplastic transformation in the P+ clonal lines of the JB6 mouse preneoplastic epidermal cells. The cloning strategy involved the use of sib selection, or screening, by pools using a biological activity assay at each subdivision of the active pool(s). The biological activity assay consisted of calcium phosphate-DNA transfection into JB6 P- recipient cells followed by determination of TPA-induced anchorage-independent colonies. A subgenomic size-selected library (3 to 12 kilobases) of BglII fragments (shown not to destroy the *pro* activity) of Cl 22 DNA was constructed by ligation into the pCD-X vector of Okayma and Berg.[67,72] Five cycles of sib selection yielded two recombinant plasmids designated p26 and p40 that contained the activated *pro* genes, *pro*-1 and *pro*-2, respectively.[72] The two active plasmids contained different sequences, as shown by lack of heteroduplex formation,[73] differences in restriction maps,[72] and absence of sequence homology.[73] Protein homology, however, may be possible since both *pro* genes appear to provide the transfected P⁻ cells with an apparently similar ability to become transformed after TPA treatment.

The structural features of the *pro*-1 gene recently sequenced[72] are unusual. The gene is relatively small (1 kb) and is principally composed of inverted complements of known mouse repeated sequences. The *pro*-1 sequence appears as a fusion of the BAM 5 and the Alu-type B1 middle repetitive elements joined by a unique sequence of 64 bp. This sequence has all the consensus sequences needed for transcription by eukaryotic RNA polymerase II. The promoter elements including a "CAAT" box, an SV-40 type core enhancer, a "TATA" box, a cap site, and a strong ribosomal binding site, are in an ordered arrangement characteristic for pol II promoters. A polyadenylation signal hexanucleotide, "ATTAAA", present in 12% of mRNAs, along with a typical cleavage site, is found in the sequence downstream to the translation terminator codon. The open reading frame of 195 bp is intronless. The predicted product of the *pro*-1 gene is a 65 amino acid protein (MW 7, 100 daltons) containing 35% hydrophobic amino acids, 24% of uncharged polar amino acids, and has a neutral isoelectric point. No significant homology between the expected *pro*-1 protein and all vertebrate protein sequences in the Georgetown Protein Bank was found.[72]

The genomic DNA segment representing the *pro*-2 gene is 3.8 kb in size and is a unique sequence except for a small highly repeated element present in the middle of the active gene.[73] This repeated element is unrelated to known mouse repeated sequences. Sequencing of the entire 3.8-kb active genomic fragment representing the *pro*-2 gene is now nearly complete.

The apparent involvement of the *pro* genes in promotion of transformation prompted Lerman and co-workers to search for possible homology to cloned viral and cellular oncogenes. Hybridization showed that neither gene is homologous to 12 known viral oncogenes: *abl, fes, fms, erb-A, erb-B, myb, myc, Ha-ras, Ki-ras, sis, src,* and mouse *c-mos*.[72,73] Sequence comparisons of the *pro*-1 sequence and the *pro*-2 sequence failed to reveal any homology to all reported oncogene sequences. Analysis of the restriction maps of both *pro* genes showed that they differ from those of *N-ras, B-lym, T-lym, N-myc, raf/mil/mht, met,* and *mcf*.[72] It thus appears likely that the *pro* genes are unrelated to known oncogenes. Because the *pro* genes act in concert with tumor promoters to bring about neoplastic transformation, they may represent a novel class of oncogenes.

Southern analyses of human and mouse genomic DNAs have demonstrated the presence of both *pro* genes, indicating their conservation during human evolution.[72] Human placenta showed both *pro*-1 and *pro*-2 homologs present in single or low copy number. Lerman et al.[74] also observed that DNA from human nasopharyngeal carcinoma cell lines contained *pro*-1 and *pro*-2 homologs. These carcinoma cell DNAs transferred promotion sensitivity when transfected into mouse JB6 P⁻ cells, suggesting that *pro* genes may be involved in human cancer induction.

The transformation-promoting activity of the *pro*-genes so far has been detected only by transfection into JB6 P⁻ cell lines. Transfection into NIH 3T3 cells or secondary mouse keratinocytes did not transfer a P⁺ response.[71-73] On the other hand, transfection of *pro* genes into human cancer-prone basal cell nevus syndrome fibroblast cells produced an extended lifespan.[75] Either *pro*-1 or *pro*-2 could independently induce the P⁺ phenotype with a specific activity similar to that of intact P⁺ DNA (Table 2).

Table 2

P+ ACTIVITY OF *PRO*-1 AND *PRO*-2 CLONED
GENES AND GENOMIC DNAs

DNA	P+ specific activity[a]
Genomic DNAs	
JB6 Cl 22	120
JB6 Cl 30	<1
Balb/c secondary mouse keratinocytes	<1
Balb/c mouse liver	<1
Human placenta	<1
Plasmids	
p26 (*pro*-1)	101
pBH (subclone of *pro*-1)	152
p40 (*pro*-2)	80
pCC3.8 (subclone of *pro*-2)	117

Note: P+ specific activity was determined from a concentration-re-
sponse curve in which TPA-induced agar colony formation
was assayed after transfection with 10^{-12} to 10^{-19} moles *pro*
gene equivalents (10 μg to 1 pg plasmid DNA) per dish of JB6
Cl 30 P− recipient cells. Genomic DNAs were assayed at 15
μg (2×10^{-17} moles) per dish (2×10^5 cells) of Cl 30 recipient
cells.

[a] TPA-induced colonies per 10^5 cells per 10^{-17} moles *pro* gene
equivalent dish.

B. *pro* Genes: Mode of Activation, Transcription, and Proposed Functions

The discovery of *pro* gene involvement in promotion of transformation and their
highly conserved nature raises further questions: (1) what distinguishes an active from
an inactive *pro* gene?, (2) what are the structures and functions of *pro* gene products?,
and (3) how do *pro* genes interact with transforming genes? Presently we have only
partial answers to these questions. One mechanism by which oncogenes become activated involves overproduction of an apparently normal oncogene product which, in
some way, perturbs normal cellular regulation and drives abnormal growth.[76,77] This
overproduction could arise from oncogene amplification, promoter activation through
gene rearrangements or viral insertions, or both. Another mechanism involves structural alteration such as point mutations in the gene and its products, presumably leading to an altered activity or regulatability of the product.[77] The lack of transformation-
promoting activity in all normal mouse and human DNAs tested, and also in the JB6
P− cell DNA (Table 2) suggests that the *pro* genes found in JB6 P+ cells (and TPA-
transformed derivatives of P+ cells) are somehow activated. Our current hypothesis is
that both elevated expression and structural alteration may be used to activate the
transformation-promoting potential of the *pro* genes. No rearrangement or significant
amplification of *pro*-2 sequence was observed in the DNA of either the P+ cell lines[72]
or mice sensitive to tumor promotion (Figure 1). Such analysis of the *pro*-1 gene in
mouse P+ and tumor cells was not possible due to its repeated sequence homology.
Both P+ and P− cells treated with TPA respond with a transient increase in cytoplasmic
RNA hybridizing to *pro*-1[72] (Table 3); this response is higher in P+ cells, suggesting
that overproduction of the gene product may occur. Also, probing the chromosomal
structure of *pro* genes has shown that the *pro* genes probably exist in transcriptionally
active chromatin.[73] These results suggest that a small structural change altering the
gene product may explain the transformation-promoting potential of the *pro*-2 gene

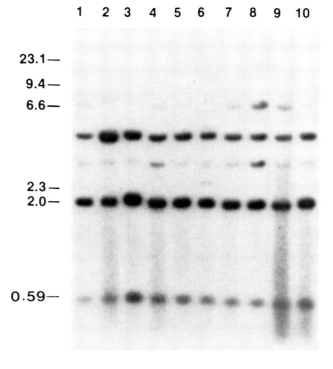

1. CI41 (cell line)
2. CI30 (cell line)
3. Sencar (liver)
4. C57/BL (liver)
5. DBA (liver)
6. BALB/c (liver)
7. JB8 (cell line)
8. D11a (cell line)
9. RT101 (cell line)
10. T-cell lymphoma (cell line)

FIGURE 1. Promotion sensitivity is not accounted for by amplification or rearrangement of the *pro*-2 gene in mouse cells. Total
DNA was digested with EcoRI to completion, electrophoresed on
1% agarose gels, and transferred to nitrocellulose filters; the filters
were hybridized under stringent conditions as described; the probe
was a 3.2-kb sequence from the 3.8-kb *pro*-2 gene.[72]

while *pro*-1 may be activated by both alteration and overproduction. Direct comparison of the DNA sequences of normal and activated alleles will be needed to demonstrate the changes responsible for the activation of *pro* genes.

What are the functions of *pro* genes? Studies on the biochemical responses to TPA
that distinguish JB6 P⁺ from P⁻ cells[48,67] have revealed a P⁺-specific decrease in synthesis of ganglioside G_7[78] and a P⁺-specific prolonged decrease in superoxide dismutase[48]
activity. Enzymes or other regulators of these events might be candidates for *pro* gene
products. The *pro* gene products may function to "switch on" the recently described[79]
novel transforming activity found in the DNA of TPA-transformed P⁺ derivatives.

Table 3
TPA TREATMENT OF BOTH P⁺ AND
P⁻ CELLS PRODUCES ELEVATION OF
PRO-1 RNA LEVELS

Cell line	pro-1 Hybridizing copies per cell	
	In untreated controls	In TPA-treated cells (2 hr)
JB6 Cl 22 (P⁺)	36 ± 9	162 ± 18
JB6 Cl 30 (P⁻)	17 ± 6	59 ± 13

Note: Levels of cytoplasmic RNA that hybridized to a *pro*-1 probe containing nucleotides 1-677 of *pro*-1[72] were determined by dot blot analysis. Results are given as the mean number of *pro*-1 copies ± half the range for two independent experiments in which cells were exposed to TPA (10 ng/mℓ; 1.6×10^{-8} *M)* for 2 hr.

IV. GENETICS OF TUMOR PROMOTION: SOME CONCLUSIONS AND UNANSWERED QUESTIONS

What follows is a consideration of insights gained into genetic determinants of sensitivity to tumor promotion, and some important unresolved issues.

A. What Genes Determine Sensitivity to Tumor Promotion?; What Functions do they Specify?

The results described earlier have made it clear that a dominantly acting single gene can confer sensitivity to promotion of neoplastic transformation by phorbol esters or various hormones. This gene can be an activated *onc* gene such as *H-ras* or one of several genes known to confer an "immortalizing" function such as *c-* or *v-myc*, pyLT, or Ad5 E1a; or this gene can be one of the recently described promotion sensitivity or *pro* genes which shows no homology to any known *onc* gene or other gene at the DNA level. It is of interest that *v-myc* transfers promotion sensitivity to JB6 promotion-insensitive cells with the same specific activity as *pro* genes.[88]

Can the promotion sensitivity function consist of immortalization? Probably not. Numerous spontaneously immortalized cell lines including mouse 3T3, 10T$_{1/2}$, and prepromotable (prepassage 35) JB6 cells, are not promotion sensitive.[64,67] Likewise, the promotion sensitivity function(s) appears not to simply consist of resistance to terminal differentiation. Differentiation-resistant putatively initiated keratinocyte cell lines have not as yet been demonstrated to be promotion sensitive. Perhaps a clonal subpopulation of these cells will turn out to be promotable.

The promotion sensitivity found in mice sensitive to initiation-promotion carcinogenesis appears to be consistently associated with a sustained epidermal hyperplasia response to tumor promoters. The promotion sensitivity found in JB6 P⁺ cells is consistently associated with a decreased synthesis of ganglioside G$_T$ and a decreased activity of the superoxide anion-removing enzyme superoxide dismutase. Both of these biochemical responses are dissociable from mitogenic response. Either of these might function as signal transducers for modulating gene expression. As for the function(s) (related to promotion sensitivity) specified by activated *H-ras*, immortalization is probably not involved, since with few exceptions,[80] immortalization or establishment appears not to be achieved with this gene. Whether any adenylate cyclase modulation via "G" proteins is involved is not clear.[81]

B. Are Initiators and Promotors Acting on the Same or Different Genetic Loci when they Produce Changes Involved in the Process of Preneoplastic Progression?

The central dogma of tumor promotion in the past has held that promotion works only on initiated cells, not on normal or near-normal cells, which show only transient responses to tumor promoters. This suggested the possibility that tumor promoters might regulate the expression of genes mutated during the initiation event to produce preneoplastic progression. Several recent findings call for a re-examination of this assumption. The finding that mice bred for sensitivity to initiation-promotion skin carcinogenesis have apparently been bred specifically for promotion sensitivity suggests that a gene for promotion sensitivity can be inherited independently of whether there exists an activated "initiation" gene. (Even if during the breeding the epidermis contained cells with activated "initiation" genes, such genes would not be inherited in the germ line.) If promotion-sensitivity genes can be inherited independently of the presence of activated initiation genes, this suggests the possibility of two (or more) separate genetic loci. Another line of evidence suggesting separate genetic loci is that reported by Furstenberger et al.[82] that first-stage tumor promotion can be achieved before — even 6 weeks before — initiation.

Recent evidence on gene cooperation[83,84] in transformation suggests (1) that two or more separate genes can cooperate or complement each other to produce a tumor cell, and (2) that there is not an obligatory sequence for events that add up to neoplastic transformation. These experiments include the demonstration that *myc* and activated *H-ras* oncogenes can function together, but not separately, to transform embryo fibroblasts after transfection.[83] The *myc* function can alternatively be provided by other genes that share with *myc* "immortalizing" activity such as adenovirus E1a or pyLT. However, this activated *ras*-complementing activity for transformation appears not to be identical to immortalizing activity. If these cooperating genes specify initiating and promoting events, respectively, in these cells, then separate loci are clearly involved.

A final suggestion for a "separate gene-nonobligatory sequence" mechanism has been set forth by Zur Hausen and co-workers,[85,86] who suggest that one route to cervical carcinoma in women involves expression of herpes virus sequences as initiators and of certain human papilloma virus genes as promoters. The herpes virus expression produces DNA alterations that are characteristic of responses specifically elicited by chemical carcinogens, not tumor promoters, and can be complemented to produce carcinomas by various agents known to show tumor-promoting activity, such as certain hormones.[85] Frequently the papilloma virus expression occurs prior to the herpes virus expression,[85,86] suggesting that a constitutively promoted state can be attained independently of initiation and there may not be an obligatory sequence of events.

REFERENCES

1. Burns, F. J., Vanderlaan, M., Snyder, E., and Albert, R. E., Induction and progression kinetics of mouse skin papillomas, in *Carcinogenesis*, Vol. 2, *Mechanisms of Tumor Promotion and Cocarcinogenesis*, Slaga, T. J., Sivak, A., and Boutwell, R. K., Eds., Raven Press, New York, 1978, 91.
2. DiGiovanni, J., Prichett, W. P., Decina, P. C., and Diamond, L., DBA/2 mice are as sensitive as Sencar mice to skin tumor promotion by 12-O-tetradecanoylphorbol-13-acetate, *Carcinogenesis*, 5, 1493, 1984.

3. Boutwell, R. K., Some biological aspects of skin carcinogenesis, *Prog. Exp. Tumor Res.*, 4, 207, 1964.
4. Reiners, J., Davidson, K., Nelson, K., Mamrack, M., and Slaga, T., Skin tumor promotion: a comparative study of several stocks and strains of mice, in *Organs and Species Specificity in Chemical Carcinogenesis*, Vol. 24, Lagenbach, R., Nesnow, S., and Rice, J. M., Eds., Plenum Press, New York, 1983, 173.
5. Strickland, J. E. and Strickland, A. G., Host cell reactivation studies with epidermal cells of mice sensitive and resistant to carcinogenesis, *Cancer Res.*, 44, 893, 1984.
6. Kinsella, A. R. and Gainer, H. St. C., In vitro studies of the possible mechanisms whereby tumour promoters mediate their responses, in *Cellular Interactions by Environmental Tumor Promoters*, Fujiki, H., Ed., Tokyo/VNU Science Press, Utrecht, 1984, 261.
7. Hecker, E., Cocarcinogenic principles from the seed oil of *Croton tiglium* and from other Euphorbiaceae, *Cancer Res.*, 28, 2338, 1968.
8. van Duuren, B. L., Tumor-promoting agents in two-stage-carcinogenesis, *Prog. Exp. Tumor Res.*, 11, 31, 1969.
9. Driedger, P. E. and Blumberg, P. M., Specific binding of phorbol ester tumor promoters, *Proc. Natl. Acad. Sci. U.S.A.*, 77, 567, 1980.
10. Pruss, R. M. and Herschman, H. R., Variants of 3T3 cells lacking mitogenic response to epidermal growth factor, *Proc. Natl. Acad. Sci. U.S.A.*, 74, 3918, 1977.
11. Pollet, R. J. and Levey, G. S., Principles of membrane receptor physiology and their application to clinical medicine, *Ann. Intern. Med.*, 92, 663, 1980.
12. Colburn, N. H., Gindhart, T. D., Hegamyer, G. A., Blumberg, P. M., Delclos, K. B., Magun, B. E., and Lockyer, J., Phorbol diester and epidermal growth factor receptors in 12-O-tetradecanoylphorbol-13-acetate-resistant and -sensitive mouse epidermal cells, *Cancer Res.*, 42, 3093, 1982.
13. Colburn, N. H., Gindhart, T. D., Dalal, B., and Hegamyer, G. A., The role of phorbol ester receptor binding in responses to promoters by mouse and human cells, in *Organ and Species Specificity in Chemical Carcinogenesis*, Vol. 24, Langenbach, R., Nesnow, S., and Rice, J. M., Eds., Plenum Press, New York, 1983, 189.
14. Fisher, P. B., Cogan, U., Horowitz, A. D., Schacter, D., and Weinstein, B., TPA resistance in friend erythroleukemia cells: role of membrane lipid fluidity, *Biochem. Biophys. Res. Commun.*, 100, 370, 1981.
15. Solanki, T. J., Slaga, M., Callahan, R., and Huberman, E., Down regulation of specific binding of [20-^{3}H]phorbol 12,13-dibutyrate and phorbol ester induced differentiation of human promyelocytic leukemia cells, *Proc. Natl. Acad. Sci. U.S.A.*, 78, 1722, 1981.
16. Collins, M. K. L. and Rozengurt, E., Homologous and heterologous mitogenic desensitization of Swiss 3T3 cells to phorbol esters and vasopressin: role of receptor and postreceptor steps, *J. Cell. Physiol.*, 118, 133, 1984.
17. Yamasaki, H., Enomoto, T., Hamel, E., and Kanno, Y., Membrane interaction and modulation of gene expression by tumor promoters, in *Cellular Interactions by Environmental Tumor Promoters*, Fujiki, H., Ed., Tokyo/VNU Science Press, Utrecht, 1984, 221.
18. Aschendel, C. L., Staller, H. M., and Boutwell, R. K., Protein kinase activity associated with a phorbol ester receptor purified from mouse brain, *Cancer Res.*, 43, 4333, 1983.
19. Kikkawa, U., Takai, Y., Tanaka, Y., Miyake, R., and Nishizuka, Y., Protein kinase C as a possible receptor protein of tumor-promoting phorbol esters, *J. Biol. Chem.*, 258, 11442, 1983.
20. Niedel, J. E., Kuhn, L. J., and Vandenbark, G. R., Phorbol diester receptor copurifies with protein kinase C, *Proc. Natl. Acad. Sci. U.S.A.*, 80, 36, 1983.
21. Gindhart, T. D., Nakamura, Y., Stevens, L. A., Hegamyer, G. A., West, M. W., Smith, B. M., and Colburn, N. H., Genes and signal transduction in tumor promotion: conclusions from studies with promoter resistant variants of JB6 mouse epidermal cells, in *Tumor Promotion and Enhancement in the Etiology of Human and Experimental Respiratory Tract Cocarcinogenesis*, Mass, M., Ed., Raven Press, New York, 1985, 341.
22. Malkison, A. M., Conway, K., Bartlett, S., Butley, M. S., and Conroy, C., Strain differences among inbred mice in protein kinase C activity, *Biochem. Biophys. Res. Commun.*, 122, 492, 1984.
23. Albert, K. A., Helmer-Matyjek, E., Nairn, A. C., Muller, T. H., Haycock, J. W., Greene, L. A., Goldstein, M., and Greengard, P., Calcium/phospholipid-dependent protein kinase (protein kinase C) phosphorylates and activates tyrosine hydroxylase, *Proc. Natl. Acad. Sci. U.S.A.*, 81, 7713, 1984.
24. Cochet, C., Gill, G. N., Meisenhelder, J., Cooper, J. A., and Hunter, T., C-kinase phosphorylates the epidermal growth factor receptor and reduces its epidermal growth factor-stimulated tyrosine protein kinase activity, *J. Biol. Chem.*, 259, 2553, 1984.
25. Iwashita, S. and Fox, C. F., Epidermal growth factor and potent phorbol tumor promoters induce epidermal growth factor receptor phosphorylation in a similar but distinctively different manner in human epidermoid carcinoma A431 cells, *J. Biol. Chem.*, 259, 2559, 1984.

Table 3

NONRANDOM NUMERICAL CHROMOSOME CHANGES IN HUMAN LEUKEMIA, LYMPHOMA, AND CANCER

Chromosome	Condition
−5	Secondary leukemia
−7	Secondary leukemia, preleukemia with infection
+7	Cancer of large bowel, bladder cancer, lymphoma
+8	ANLL, blastic phase of CML, polyps of colon, preleukemia
−9	Bladder cancer
+12	CLL, seminoma, lymphocytic lymphoma
+19	Blastic phase of CML
+21	ALL
−22	Meningioma, sarcoma
+22	ANLL

Table 4

NONRANDOM TRANSLOCATIONS CHARACTERIZING HUMAN CANCERS

Translocation	Condition
t(3;8)(p25;q21)	Mixed tumor of parotid
t(6;14)(q21;q24)	Serous cystadenocarcinoma of ovary
t(11;22)(q24;q12)	Ewing's sarcoma, Peripheral neuroepithelioma (neuroblastoma)
t(12;16)(q13;q11)	Liposarcoma
t(x;18)(p11;q11)	Synovial sarcoma

Table 5

NONRANDOM MORPHOLOGIC AND NUMERICAL CHROMOSOME CHANGES IN HUMAN CANCER

Chromosome	Condition
1p-(p34)	Neuroblastoma
1p-(p11p22)	Malignant melanoma
1p-(p31p36)	Neuroblastoma
1p-,i(1q)	Endometrial cancer
1q+,1p-(qter-p21)	Breast cancer
1q+(q24q44?)	Large bowel cancer
1q+	Breast cancer
3p-(p14p23)	Small cell cancer of lung
3p-	Renal cancer
3q+	Nasopharyngeal cancer
i(5p)	Bladder cancer
5q-,+7,−9	Cervical cancer
6q-(q11q31),i(6p)	Malignant melanoma
i(6p)	Retinoblastoma
6q-(q15)	Ovarian cancer
8q-(q11q22)	Salivary gland tumors
11p-(p13)	Wilms tumor
11q-	Cervical cancer
i(12p)	Seminoma, teratoma
12q-(q22q24)	Large bowel cancer
12q-(q13q15)	Salivary gland tumors
13q-(q14),-13	Retinoblastoma
22q-(q11),-22	Meningioma

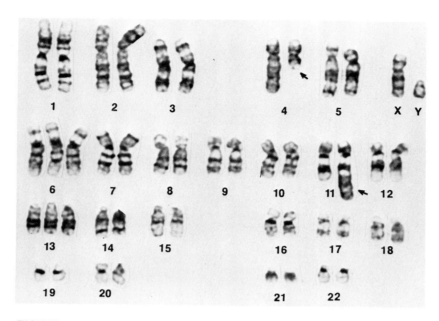

FIGURE 3. Specific chromosomal change, t(4;11)(q11;q32), characterizing a subgroup of cases with ALL. The disease with this translocation is usually lymphoblastic in nature, but may be associated with myelomonocytic features. Generally, it carries a poor prognosis.

somes in the compact environment of the interphase nucleus. Inasmuch as the histologic morphology of the nuclei varies from tissue to tissue, and in fact is utilized by cytologists and pathologists in the recognition of specific cells and tissues, there must be a definite architectural orientation system followed by the chromosomes in different cell types. Whether the specific location of the chromosomes is the same in all human nuclei, or whether there are differences which account for nuclear morphologic variability in tissues, is an area certainly deserving the closest attention and investigation. Since certain karyotypic events associated with malignancy occur with a high consistency, it would seem to imply that there is an order which the chromosomes must obey (including their location and orientation in interphase nuclei) if we are to explain these recurring events and their meaning in carcinogenesis.

IV. CHROMOSOME CHANGES IN NEOPLASIA: THEIR NATURE AND EFFECTS

There is little doubt that the chromosome changes play a role in carcinogenesis. What has to be clarified is whether such changes are the basic events leading to malignant transformation, or whether they are a secondary phenomenon, however crucial they may be in the biology of the neoplastic process. It would appear that the demonstration of recurring and consistent karyotypic events in certain human neoplastic entities (Figure 3 and 4) speaks for a basic cause which is responsible for these events, and thus, one must seek such a cause beyond the karyotypic phenomena. What is possible is that once the basic cause has led to the genesis of karyotypic changes, the latter are necessary for malignant transformation to occur.[7] Though this may sound like a very sweeping statement, it is difficult, at least in human neoplastic conditions, to find a leukemic or cancerous entity which is not accompanied by abnormal chromosomal manifestations. There are those who point to the demonstration that certain

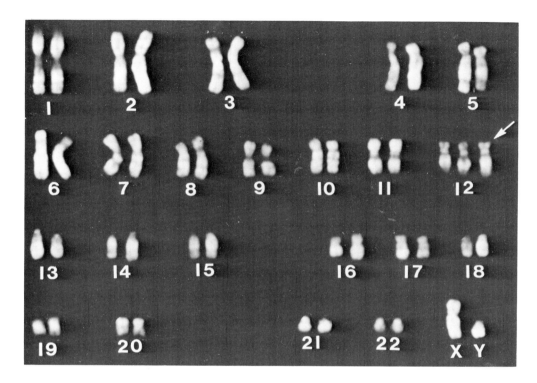

FIGURE 4. Characteristic chromosomal change, i.e., trisomy 12 (+12), in CLL. This change affects a substantial number of cases with this disease.

tumors or leukemias are characterized primarily by normal (diploid) karyotypes. However, in these cases one cannot be sure that these diploid cells have not originated from normal supportive cells or contaminating leukocytes, or rule out the possibility that a submicroscopic karyotypic event may have occurred, sufficient onto itself to cause the neoplasia. In most, if not the preponderant, number of human leukemias and cancers, the affected cells are characterized by a primary cytogenetic event which is related to, or at least associated with, the process of malignant transformation;[8-10] such primary events have been listed in Tables 1 through 5. What complicates the cytogenetic picture further is the fact that the primary karyotypic event is almost invariably accompanied by additional chromosomal changes which can vary from a few to numerous and complex ones, including those of numerical and/or morphological nature.[11] The role of the additional chromosome changes in the carcinogenetic process has not received as much attention as that of the primary karyotypic change, though in my opinion they may bear more directly on the sum of the manifestations of neoplasia than is presently realized (Figure 5). Furthermore, it is my opinion that a neoplastic process is at its lowest level of malignancy when characterized only by the primary karyotypic change, and that such manifestations as increases in proliferative activity, drug sensitivity, tumor invasiveness, metastatic spread, and aggressiveness are more likely to be directly related to the additional chromosome changes than to the primary karyotypic event.

V. CHROMOSOME CHANGES AND ONCOGENES

The primary karyotypic change can assume one of a number of forms: translocation, deletion, insertion, inversion, addition, and numerical variation (a missing or extra

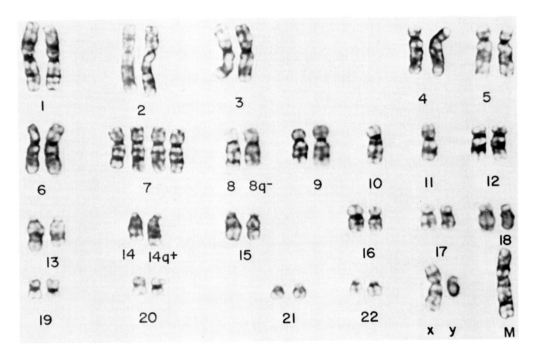

FIGURE 5.   Karyotype of a cell from a patient with BL showing the 8;14 translocation described in Figure 8. In addition to this primary (specific) chronosomal change, a number of secondary changes, i.e., +7, +7, −10, −11, and a marker, was present. These changes may play a crucial role in the biology of the tumor and possibly in the differences in the clinical manifestations seen in endemic and nonendemic BL (see text).

chromosome). Particular attention has been given in recent years to translocations which are reciprocal and balanced in nature, i.e., a karyotypic event in which there is no loss of chromosomal (or DNA) material during an exchange of segments between two or more chromosomes. Often under these circumstances, involvement of proto-oncogenes, as well as translocation of oncogenes and their activation, may take place.[4,5] A number of these cellular oncogenes has been characterized through their relationship to sequences of oncogenes carried by retroviruses, i.e., there appears to be considerable homology in the nucleic acid make-up of some of the oncogenes associated with such translocations (c-oncogenes) and those characterizing oncogenes carried by retroviruses (v-oncogenes).[12-14] An example of a translocation affecting a proto-oncogene is the one alluded to earlier, i.e., the Ph translocation in human chronic myelocytic leukemia (CML).[1] During this cytogenetic event, breaks occur in chromosome 9 at band q34, and another in chromosome 22 at band q11, leading to deletions and exchanges of material between these two chromosomes (Figure 6). Since the amount of chromosomal material lost by chromosome 22 is larger than that which it obtains from chromosome 9, it leads to an abbreviated chromosome which is readily recognized in unbanded and banded preparations, known as the "Ph chromosome". Molecularly, the Ph translocation results in the transfer of material from the proto-oncogene *abl* present on the long arm of chromosome 9 at band q34 *(c-abl),* to the abbreviated long arm of chromosome 22 at band q11, contiguous with part of a possible gene (*bcr*) present on chromosome 22.[15-17] Recent evidence indicates that the messenger RNA (mRNA) expressed by this translocated oncogene, possibly in conjunction with *bcr*, is of a different nature than that observed in normal cells, i.e., the normal mRNA produced by *c-abl* is 6 to 7 kb, whereas the abnormal one, resulting from the

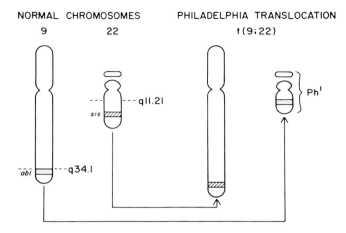

FIGURE 6.   Schematic presentation of events leading to the genesis of the Ph chromosome. The break on chromosome 9 is at band q34.1 and apparently involves the oncogene *abl* which is then translocated to the abbreviated chromosome 22, which has been deleted at band q11.21. The material from chromosome 22 is translocated to chromosome 9, and included in it is the oncogene *sis*. In CML, *sis* may or may not be activated, but does not appear to be expressed as a result of the Ph translocation.

Ph translocation, is 8 to 9 kb.[18-20] Thus, this is one of the few existing demonstrations that a gene involved in a chromosomal translocation may produce mRNA which is different in nature than that of the gene in normal cells. The possibility exists that such abnormal mRNA may lead to the production of abnormal proteins, which may possibly be involved in the direct causation of the CML. Incidentally, another cellular oncogene (*sis*), which is translocated with the material from chromosome 22 onto the long arm of chromosome 9, is often not activated, inasmuch as the cytogenetic events do not directly affect band 22q12 at which this oncogene is located.[21]

To demonstrate the usefulness and sensitivity of these molecular approaches, variant Ph translocations may serve as an appropriate example.[1,22] These variant Ph translocations had been divided on cytologic basis into two varieties: the *simple* variety which involves chromosome 22 (which invariably constitutes the Ph chromosome) in a translocation with a chromosome other than 9, and the *complex* variety of Ph translocations in which (though chromosome 9 is often involved) a number of chromosomes may be involved in a Ph translocation (Figure 7). Before molecular probes were available, it was thought that chromosome 9 often escaped being involved in such variant Ph translocations, particularly of the simple variety. However, recent evidence points to a strong possibility that a translocation of the oncogene *abl* to the Ph chromosome always takes place,[23] with the possibility that the oncogene *abl* is thus activated and appears to be consistently involved in the cytogenetic events related to CML. The break on chromosome 22 at band q11 leading to the Ph occurs within a relatively small area of only several kbs, and is called *bcr*,[15] which appears to be directly involved in the process of translocation with the oncogene *abl*. In fact, it appears that part of *bcr* remaining on chromosome 22 interacts with the oncogene *abl* and creates a new gene which may be responsible for the abnormal mRNAs mentioned earlier.

The specificity and sensitivity of molecular probes is reflected in recent results regarding events on chromosome 22, in particular at band q11. By utilizing appropriate probes for light-chain immunoglobulins (λ) on this chromosome, it has been demon-

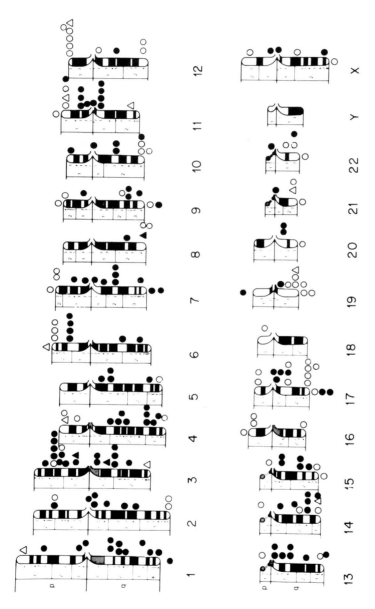

FIGURE 7.   Chromosome bands involved in variant Ph translocations. Only the Y chromosome has not been described to be affected by such an event, with every other chromosome having been involved in either simple (open circles) or complex (solid circles) Ph translocations. Triangles indicate acute leukemias which were Ph positive. As can be seen, breaks on the chromosomes involved in variant Ph translocations affect almost every oncogene location, possibly leading to their activation (see text).

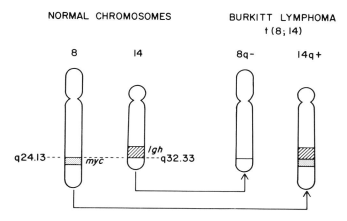

FIGURE 8.   Schematic presentation of events occurring during the translocation seen in BL, i.e., t(8; 14)(q24; q32). As can be seen, the break on chromosome 8 appears to affect the oncogene *myc* which is then translocated to chromosome 14 in apposition to the genes for heavy immunoglobulins (Igh).

strated that the gene for the constant region of λ is translocated *in toto* during t(8;22) in Burkitt lymphoma (BL), and that it remains *in toto* on chromosome 22 in CML during t(9;22), but is split with part remaining on 22 and part being translocated to 9; in some cases of ALL with t(9;22).[24] Thus, it appears that even Ph chromosomes which in the past were thought to be identical in their genesis as based on cytologic evidence, may have a variable composition as demonstrated with molecular probes.

Another balanced and reciprocal translocation which has been studied intensively is that seen frequently in BL, in which breaks occur on chromosome 8 at band q34 and chromosome 14 at band q24[1] (Figure 8). In the process of translocation, not only are various heavy-chain immunoglobulin genes affected (these have been related to several facets of the malignant lymphoma), but also activation and overexpression of the oncogene *myc* occur.[25-27] In contrast to the situation in CML associated with an abnormal mRNA as a result of the Ph translocation, no qualitative differences have been demonstrated in the mRNA as a result of the *myc* translocation, though quantitative differences do exist. Whether this quantitative difference in the product by the oncogene *myc* can account for and/or play a role in carcinogenesis (in this case BL and other lymphomas) has not been established. What appears essential is to expand such studies to other conditions associated with translocations or other karyotypic events known to affect the loci of various oncogenes, and to relate the expression and products of such oncogenes to the conditions under study.

Complicating the studies on oncogene activation and expression is the fact that often the primary karyotypic event affecting an oncogene is subsequently followed by activation and expression of varying numbers of oncogenes, leading to an array of their products.[28-30] The challenge resides in deciphering not only which of these products are essential for the process of carcinogenesis, but also which are of normal and abnormal expression, and which are temporary or permanent. This challenge will require close correlation with the karyotypic events, since there is a strong possibility that those oncogene expressions which are permanent may be related to chromosomal changes, whereas temporary oncogene activation may be a manifestation either of normal cellular function or temporary activation of proto-oncogenes.

Table 6
CHROMOSOME ONCOGENE
LOCATIONS IN THE HUMAN
GENOME

Chromosome	Location	Oncogene
1	1p32	c-Blym-1
1	1p13-p22	c-N-ras
1	1q12-qter	c-sk
2	2p21-23	N-myc
3	3p25	c-raf-1
4		c-raf-2
5	5q34	c-fms
6	6q23-q12	c-K-ras 1
6	6q22-24	c-myb
7	7p11-13	c-erb B
8	8q22	c-mos
8	8q24	c-myc
9	9q34.1	c-abl
11	11p15	c-H-ras 1
11	11q13	bcl-1
11	11q23-24	c-ets
12	12p12	c-K-ras 2
12	12pter-q14	c-int
14	14q21-q31	c-fos
15	15q26.1	c-fes
17	17p12-q21	c-erb A
18	18q21	bcl-2
18		c-erv-1
20	20q12-q13	s-src
22	22q13.1	c-sis
X		c-H-ras 2

VI. HOW MANY ONCOGENES?

Though several dozen oncogenes have been identified (and for most of them, chromosomal locations ascertained — Table 6), we know the nature of the products of only a few, and little about the effects of their products on cells; particularly the role they play in carcinogenesis. If one subscribes to the concept and significance of the primary karyotypic event as a key for malignant transformation, it is possible, if not likely, that many more oncogenes exist than is presently realized, and that the nature of these oncogenes and their role in carcinogenesis will require further refinement of techniques for their identification. It is tempting to state that since the human may be subject to several hundred specific neoplastic states, several hundred oncogenes exist. In fact, one of the contributions of cytogenetics to oncology (and carcinogenesis) has been the demonstration that clinical entities which appeared to be cytologically, biochemically, clinically, and prognostically similar, have been shown to consist of a number of subentities on the basis of the primary chromosome event. This has been particularly true in the leukemias, though similar observations are now being extended to solid tumors, e.g., those of the bladder. In the latter cancer,[31] we have been able to demonstrate that cytogenetically at least three subentities of transitional cell carcinoma of the bladder and related tissues exist, with each being characterized by a specific karyotypic event, i.e., an isochromosome of the short arm of chromosome 5 [i(5p)], monosomy 9 and trisomy 7. Whether these specific karyotypic changes point to a possibility that each entity is due to a separate etiologic agent, or whether they represent variations, possibly at the molecular level of the transitional cell population of the bladder (and other tissues), is an area which will require future investigation.

Events associated with chromosome loss or the acquisition of extra chromosomes may reflect a homozygous situation in which certain genes can be activated and, thus, lead to the carcinogenetic process. Evidence in this direction is rather scarce, and activation of known oncogenes through partial or complete monosomy or trisomy has not been clearly established to date.

It appears from the earlier discussion that activation of genes possibly responsible for the process of carcinogenesis, or at least necessary for its manifestations, may appear in several cytogenetic guises. The effects of translocations may involve the transfer of material from a proto-oncogene to a new chromosomal location, resulting in the activation of the oncogene. A similar situation may occur through insertion of a segment from another chromosome. The processes of deletion or inversion may achieve a similar result, since they tend to rearrange or modify the material within a chromosome and, thus, possibly activate existing oncogenes. The means by which extra or missing chromosomes lead to activation of cancer (or other) genes (as indicated earlier) have not been established with certainty, though the process of homozygosity (actual or effective) remains a possibility. The relationship of chromosomal breaks occurring in translocations, insertions, and inversions to common and inherited fragile sites, is an area which has received some attention recently, but one in which the last word has not been established. Sufficient exceptions exist, e.g., breaks occurring at sites in affected (leukemic) cells of patients in whom such fragile sites could not be demonstrated and vice versa, to warrant further investigation.

VII. TYPES OF CHROMOSOME CHANGES IN NEOPLASIA AND RELATION TO CARCINOGENESIS

With improvements in cytogenetic techniques, and with concerted efforts, more and more human neoplastic entities have been and will continue to be demonstrated to be characterized by primary (or specific) chromosome changes. Furthermore, cytogenetically, almost every human disease examined to date has been shown to be karyotypically abnormal and, most importantly, characterized by subentities with similar, if not identical, primary karyotypic events. Thus, the cytogenetic changes, even if they may not play a direct role in carcinogenesis, certainly reflect events which point to different mechanisms operative in the genesis of subentities within entities which, on the basis of available knowledge and approaches, were thought to be homogeneous. This cytogenetic definition of subentities has been one of the major contributions of cytogenetics to carcinogenesis, besides its important practical application in the understanding and therapy of various clinical neoplastic diseases. It is difficult to escape the contention that the presence of consistent chromosomal changes, which not only characterize specific disease entities, but also consistently involve the same submicroscopic chromosomal locus, points to the significance of these changes in the carcinogenic process.

One of the crucial questions to be answered is whether different basic mechanisms can lead to the genesis of an identical karyotypic change in a particular cell. The specificity of chromosome changes for involved cell types has already been established, with the possibility existing that such an event in other cell types may not lead to a carcinogenic process or, if it does, cell death occurs and thus prevents the affected cell from proliferating. What the chromosome changes indicate is that specific karyotypic changes must affect a particular type of cell in order for malignant transformation and proliferation to occur. Thus, the chromosomal change must hold a crucial position either in the basic mechanism leading to the malignant process and, if not, at least in the perpetuation of an abnormal proliferative capacity and behavior of cancer cells.

REFERENCES

1. Sandberg, A. A., *The Chromosomes in Human Cancer and Leukemia,* Elsevier/North-Holland, New York, 1980, 776.
2. Mitelman, F., Catalog of chromosome aberrations in cancer, *Cytogenet. Cell Genet.,* 36, 1, 1983.
3. Yunis, J. J., Comparative analysis of high-resolution chromosome techniques, *Cancer Genet. Cytogenet.,* 7, 43, 1982.
4. Bishop, M. J., Cellular oncogenes and retroviruses, *Annu. Rev. Biochem.,* 52, 301, 1983.
5. Varmus, H. E., The molecular genetics of cellular oncogenes, *Am. Rev. Genet.,* 18, 533, 1984.
6. Krontiris, T. G., The emerging genetics of human cancer, *N. Engl. J. Med.,* 309, 404, 1983.
7. Sandberg, A. A., A chromosomal hypothesis of oncogenesis, *Cancer Genet. Cytogenet.,* 8, 277, 1983.
8. Rowley, J. D., Identification of the constant chromosome regions involved in human hematologic malignant diseaes, *Science,* 216, 749, 1982.
9. Rowley, J. D. and Testa, J. R., Chromosome abnormalities in malignant hematologic diseases, *Adv. Cancer Res.,* 36, 103, 1982.
10. Sandberg, A. A., Chromosomes in human neoplasia, in *Current Problems in Cancer,* Vol. 8, No. 2, Year Book Medical, Chicago, 1983, 1.
11. Sandberg, A. A., Chromosomal changes in human cancer: specificity and heterogeneity, in *Tumor Cell Heterogeneity: Origins and Implications,* Vol. 4, Owens, A. H., Jr., Coffey, P. S., and Baylin, S. B., Eds., Academic Press, New York, 1982, 367.
12. Goff, S. P., D'Eustachio, P., Ruddle, F. H., and Baltimore, D., Chromosomal assignment of the endogenous proto-oncogene c-*abl, Science,* 218, 1317, 1982.
13. Hunter, T., Oncogenes and proto-oncogenes: how do they differ?, *J. Natl. Cancer Inst.,* 73, 773, 1984.
14. Twardzik, D. R., Todaro, G. J., Marquardt, H., Reynolds, F. E., Jr., and Stephenson, J. R., Transformation induced by Abelson murine leukemia virus involves production of a polypeptide growth factor, *Science,* 216, 894, 1982.
15. Bartram, C. R., de Klein, A., Hagemeijer, A., van Agthoven, T., Geurts van Kessel, A., Bootsma, D., Grosveld, G., Ferguson-Smith, M. A., Davies, T., Stone, M., Heisterkamp, N., Stephenson, J. R., and Groffen, J., Translocation of c-*abl* oncogene correlates with the presence of a Philadelphia chromosome in chronic myelocytic leukaemia, *Nature (London),* 306, 277, 1983.
16. Groffen, J., Stephenson, J. R., Heisterkamp, N., de Klein, A., Bartram, C. R., and Grosveld, G., Philadelphia chromosomal breakpoints are clustered within a limited region, *bcr,* on chromosome 22, *Cell,* 36, 93, 1984.
17. Bartram, C. R., Kleihauer, E., de Klein, A., Grosveld, G., Teyssier, J. R., Heisterkamp, N., and Groffen, J., C-*abl* and *bcr* rearranged in a Ph¹-negative CML patient, *EMBO J.,* 4, 683, 1985.
18. Gale, R. P. and Canaani, E., An 8 kilobase *abl* RNA transcript in chronic myelogenous leukemia, *Proc. Natl. Acad. Sci. U.S.A.,* 81, 5648, 1984.
19. Leibowitz, D., Cubbon, R., and Bank, A., Increased expression of a novel c-abl-related RNA in K562 cells, *Blood,* 65, 526, 1985.
20. Collins, S. J., Kubonishi, I., Miyoshi, I., and Groudine, M. T., Altered transcription of the c-*abl* oncogene in K-562 and other chronic myelogenous leukemia cells, *Science,* 225, 72, 1984.
21. Groffen, J., Heisterkamp, N., Stephenson, J. R., Geurts van Kessel, A., de Klein, A., Grosveld, G., and Bootsma, D., C-*sis* is translocated from chromosome 22 to chromosome 9 in chronic myelocytic leukemia, *J. Exp. Med.,* 158, 9, 1983.
22. Sandberg, A. A., Chromosomes and causation of human cancer and leukemia. XL. The Ph¹ and other translocations in CML, *Cancer,* 46, 2221, 1980.
23. Hagemeijer, A., Bartram, C. R., Smith, E. M. E., van Agthoven, A. J., and Bootsma, D., Is the chromosomal region 9q34 always involved in variants of the Ph¹ translocation?, *Cancer Genet. Cytogenet.,* 13, 1, 1984.
24. Cannizzaro, L. A., Nowell, P. C., Croce, C. M., and Emanuel, B. S., The breakpoint in 22q11 for a t(9;22) acute lymphocytic leukemia differs from the breakpoint of t(8;22) Burkitt's lymphoma, *Cancer Genet. Cytogenet.,* 18, 173, 1985.
25. Croce, C. M., Erikson, J., ar-Rushdi, A., Aden, D., and Nishikura, K., The translocated c-myc gene of Burkitt lymphoma is transcribed in plasma cells and repressed in lymphoblastoid cells, *Proc. Natl. Acad. Sci. U.S.A.,* 81, 3170, 1984.
26. Cruce, C. M., Tsujimoto, Y., Erikson, J., and Nowell, P., Biology of disease. Chromosome translocations and B cell neoplasia, *Lab. Invest.,* 51, 258, 1984.
27. Croce, C. M., Thierfelder, W., Erikson, J., Nishikura, K., Finan, J., Lenoir, G. M., and Nowell, P. C., Transcriptional activation of an unrearranged and untranslocated c-*myc* oncogene by translocation of a Cλ locus in Burkitt lymphoma cells, *Proc. Natl. Acad. Sci. U.S.A.,* 80, 6922, 1983.

28. Slamon, D. J., deKernion, J. B., Verma, I. M., and Cline, M. J., Expression of cellular oncogenes in human malignancies, *Science,* 224, 256, 1984.
29. McClain, K. L., Expression of oncogenes in human leukemias, *Cancer Res.,* 44, 5382, 1984.
30. Rosson, D. and Tereba, A., Transcription of hematopoietic-associated oncogenes in childhood leukemia, *Cancer Res.,* 43, 3912, 1983.
31. Gibas, Z., Prout, G. R., Pontes, J. E., Connolly, J. G., and Sandberg, A. A., A specific chromosome change (i5p) in transitional cell carcinoma of the bladder, *Cancer Genet. Cytogenet.,* 19, 229, 1986.

Chapter 7

DNA REACTIVE AND EPIGENETIC CARCINOGENS

Gary M. Williams

TABLE OF CONTENTS

I. INTRODUCTION

One of the most important advances in the understanding of chemical carcinogenesis came from the discovery beginning in the late 1950s that the ultimate carcinogenic form of many chemicals was a reactive electrophilic species. Major research in this area was contributed by the team of J. and E. Miller at the McArdle Laboratories, who generalized these observations into the concept that "electrophilic reactants are the active forms of most, and possibly all, carcinogens . . . ".[1] Investigations by the Millers, Brookes, Gelboin, Magee, Weisburger, and others established the principle that diverse organic carcinogens undergo biotransformation to ultimate electrophiles which can react with nucleophilic sites in a variety of cellular macromolecules, including DNA.[2,3] The recognition of the need for metabolic activation of otherwise inert procarcinogens lead researchers in the genetic field to combine mammalian enzyme preparations with prokaryotic or eukaryotic cells in culture in order to document the mutagenicity of carcinogens.[4] As a result, the pioneering observations of Auerbach and others[5] on the mutagenicity of reactive alkylating chemicals were extended to a large number of activation-dependent carcinogens.[6,7] From such findings, Ames and co-workers[6] arrived at the conclusion that "carcinogens are mutagens".

These important generalizations on electrophilicity and gene mutagenicity have proven to be true for many carcinogens. Nonetheless, for a substantial number of carcinogens, evidence of DNA-reactivity, including identification of an electrophilic derivative, positive results in short-term tests, and significant binding to DNA, has not been obtained. This led a number of scientists to consider the possibility that the many diverse types of carcinogens might operate through a variety of different mechanisms.[8-13] Indeed, Miller and Miller[14] emphasized that even with electrophilic carcinogens, both genetic and epigenetic mechanisms of carcinogenesis must be considered.

If there are any differences in the mechanisms by which chemicals induce cancer, then in principle, carcinogens can be classified according to their properties that underly specific mechanisms. In 1977, the proposal was made to distinguish between two major categories of carcinogen;[8,9] one, referred to as genotoxic, was considered to be capable of reacting with DNA, while the other, called epigenetic, was conceived to lack the property of reacting with DNA, but to exert other biological effects that were the basis of their carcinogenicity. Using available information, various carcinogens were assigned to specific classes within these two categories, while agents, for which the information required for classification was not sufficient, remained unclassified[15] (Table 1).

The concept of mechanistically different carcinogens and the classification of them have now been used by many investigators[12,13,15-19] and have received a degree of acceptance by working groups.[20-22] On the other hand, aspects of this approach have been questioned by some scientists.[23-27] The current evidence for the distinction between genotoxic and epigenetic carcinogens will be reviewed here.

II. DNA-REACTIVE (GENOTOXIC) CARCINOGENS

In the categorization of carcinogens developed by Weisburger and Williams,[15] the classical organic carcinogens which form electrophilic reactants were designated as genotoxic. The term genotoxic was originally proposed in 1973 by a working group[28] to denote toxic, lethal, and heritable effects to karyotic and extra-karyotic genetic material in germinal and somatic cells. It was proposed as a general term to describe the components of chemical interaction with genetic material. In the first few years after its introduction, the term appeared not to have been adopted by the scientific community and, therefore, it was used in the proposed categorization of carcinogens in

Table 1
CLASSIFICATION OF CARCINOGENIC CHEMICALS

Category and class	Example
DNA-reactive carcinogens	
Activation independent	Alkylating agent
Activation dependent	Polycyclic aromatic hydrocarbon, nitrosamine
Inorganic[a]	Metal
Epigenetic carcinogens	
Promoting	Organochlorine pesticides
	Saccharin
Endocrine-modifying	Estrogen
	Amitrole
Immunosuppressant	Purine analog
Cytotoxic	Nitrilotriacetic acid
Peroxisome proliferator	Clofibrate
Solid state	Plastics
Unclassified	Methapyrilene
	Dioxane

[a] Some are categorized as genotoxic because of evidence for damage of DNA; others may operate through epigenetic mechanisms such as alterations in fidelity of DNA polymerases.

1979[8,9] in a more restricted sense to specifically designate the reaction of chemicals with DNA. Subsequently, however, authors began to use "genotoxic" in several ways, including to refer to any positive effect in short-term tests. The latter current general usage does not precisely correspond to the meaning in the 1979 classification, and, therefore, the term DNA-reactive has been applied as being more specific to the description of carcinogens that undergo chemical reaction with DNA.[29]

In the categorization of a carcinogen as DNA-reactive, the only definitive proof of this property is the demonstration of the formation of adducts in DNA. Such measurements can now be made with a variety of sensitive techniques.[16,30-32] For a carcinogen with a structure compatible with the formation of an electrophile, positive results in genotoxicity assays can be substituted for DNA binding studies as evidence of DNA-reactivity, provided convincing findings are obtained in a reliable battery of tests.[33] Nevertheless, short-term tests are not the primary or the only basis on which the distinction between DNA-reactive and other types of carcinogens is made, contrary to the implications of some authors.[26,27] In particular, negative results alone are not sufficient to preclude DNA-reactivity, and when only one or a few positive results are available together with negative results, a careful analysis of all the data must be made.

In the use of short-term tests to assess DNA-reactivity, some measurements, such as those for DNA damage or DNA repair, correlate better with this property of chemicals than do other assays such as those for chromosomal effects or transformation, which may stem from actions on cellular components other than DNA.[34] Many carcinogens produce chromosome mutations,[35] but agents that produce only chromosome mutations cannot be concluded to be DNA-reactive, since chromosomal alteration can be caused by effects on the mitotic spindle, and possibly other actions.[36] For this reason, a number of chemicals can produce chromosomal alterations, but yet no specific gene changes. Even less is known about the molecular basis of transformation than is understood for chromosomal effects.[37] Transformation is produced by carcinogens that are DNA-reactive, but others that are not known to react with DNA also cause transformation.[38] Chromosome aberrations and transformation have been recommended in screening batteries to detect both DNA-reactive and epigenetic carcinogens,[33] but more

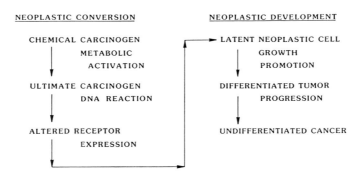

FIGURE 1.   Schematic outline of the carcinogenic processes.

detailed research on the underlying mechanisms is needed to establish the significance of these endpoints.

Findings of isolated effects in short-term tests have occasionally been taken as evidence that a chemical reacts with DNA. For example, 12-*O*-tetradecanoyl-13-phorbol acetate (TPA), the widely used active component of croton oil (a historic tool in research on the mechanisms of neoplasm promotion) has been reported to increase sister-chromatid exchanges; this has been interpreted as evidence that it is genotoxic.[25] However, several considerations dictate caution in the interpretation of positive findings in sister-chromatid exchange assays. To begin with, there is evidence that sister-chromatid exchanges are produced by the agents or conditions used to differentiate chromatids and, consequently, can be elevated by alteration of the cellular effects of these components.[39] This being the case, small increases in sister-chromatid exchanges are of questionable significance. Moreover, even the unequivocal induction of sister-chromatid exchanges is not definite evidence of DNA-reactivity,[40,41] and, therefore, such findings alone cannot be taken as proof that the chemical forms adducts with DNA. In fact, TPA has not been shown to bind to DNA. Nevertheless, it is possible that TPA may indirectly give rise to DNA damage through intracellular generation of oxygen radicals,[42] but that is a totally different action than chemical reaction of an electrophilic form of the agent itself with DNA.

To summarize, the structures of DNA-reactive carcinogens are such that they form electrophilic reactants, usually through specific metabolic reactions. As a consequence, these carcinogens, for the most part, are reliably positive in a variety of genotoxicity assays. Moreover, the exact chemical structure of the adducts in DNA has been demonstrated for many. Most of the commonly studied experimental organic carcinogens are DNA-reactive.[39-43]

The property of DNA-reactivity is very likely the actual critical effect of carcinogens of this type in producing cancer. As shown in Figure 1, the process of chemical carcinogenesis can be divided into two necessary and mechanistically distinct sequences. The first of these, neoplastic conversion, involves the generation of a neoplastic cell. Considerable evidence has accrued to support the concept that this sequence involves a genetic alteration of the cell.[29] Change in the genome can be caused in several ways, including alteration in the structure and function of DNA as a result of chemical damage. Current research has implicated cellular oncogenes as likely critical gene sequences whose altered expression could be the basis for neoplastic conversion.[44-46] Thus, DNA-reactive carcinogens probably induce neoplasia largely as a consequence of their reaction with DNA, which leads to neoplastic conversion of the affected cells. Nevertheless, DNA-reactive carcinogens also exert other cellular and tissue effects, and these could facilitate the second sequence of carcinogenesis — neoplastic development. Some

Table 2
CHARACTERISTICS OF CARCINOGENICITY OF DNA-REACTIVE CARCINOGENS

Occasionally active with single exposure
Frequently active at low (i.e., subtoxic) doses
Can have additive or synergistic effects with one another
Can be active transplacentally, and carcinogenicity often increased in neonates
Subcarcinogenic effects can be made manifest by subsequent promoting action
Effects can be enhanced by cocarcinogens
Organotropism shifted by modifiers of biotransformation

Table 3
GENOTOXICITY OF CHEMICALS JUDGED TO BE CARCINOGENIC TO HUMANS BY THE INTERNATIONAL AGENCY FOR RESEARCH ON CANCER

Chemical	Evidence for activity in short-term tests
4-Aminobiphenyl	Sufficient
Arsenic and arsenic compounds	Limited
Asbestos	Inadequate
Azathioprine	Limited
Benzene	Limited
Benzidine	Sufficient
N-N-Bis(2-chloroethyl)naphthylamine	Limited
Bis(chloromethyl)ether	Limited
Chlorambucil	Sufficient
Chromium and certain chromium compounds	Sufficient
Combined chemotherapy for lymphomas	Inadequate
Conjugated estrogens	Inadequate
Cyclophosphamide	Sufficient
Diethylstilbestrol	Inadequate
Melphalan	Sufficient
Mustard gas	Sufficient
Myleran	Sufficient
2-Naphthylamine	Sufficient
Nickel and certain nickel compounds	Inadequate
Phenacetin-containing analgesics	Limited
Soots, tars, and oils	Sufficient
Treosulphan	Inadequate
Vinyl chloride	Sufficient

of the differences in the potencies of DNA-reactive carcinogens may in fact be attributable to these nongenetic effects. As a consequence of the mode of action of DNA-reactive carcinogens, the characteristics of their carcinogenic effects in experimental systems (Table 2) are indicative of a high degree of hazard to humans. It is probably for this reason that the majority of carcinogens recognized as having caused human cancer is of the DNA-reactive type (Table 3).[47]

III. EPIGENETIC CARCINOGENS

Although many carcinogens have the property of DNA-reactivity, there is a substantial number of carcinogens whose structure, or that of their metabolites, does not suggest a likely electrophilic reactant, and which have been inactive or yielded equivocal results in short-term tests for genotoxicity.[21] The formation of adducts in DNA by such carcinogens, using sensitive techniques, has not been found. Examples include saccharin,[48] chloroform,[49] perchloroethylene,[50] trichloroethylene,[51,52] di(2-ethylhexyl)-phthalate,[53] estone, and estradiol.[17]

In addition to evidence of a lack of DNA-reactivity, such carcinogens have been demonstrated to display other primary effects not involving DNA binding, but which could account for their carcinogenicity. Effects of this type include cytotoxicity, peroxisome proliferation, neoplasm promotion, endocrine modification, and immunosuppression.[15] Carcinogens that are not DNA-reactive and have displayed another of the properties that could underlie an increase in neoplasms have been classified as epigenetic (Table 1). It is important to note that carcinogens that have not been found to be DNA-reactive, but for which an alternative effect that could be the basis of carcinogenicity has not been reasonably established, remain unclassified. That is, lack of DNA-reactivity is not sufficient for assignment to the epigenetic category. For this reason, the term ''nongenotoxic'' used by some does not correspond to the fuller meaning of the term epigenetic.

Carcinogens that do not chemically attack DNA can nevertheless produce an increase in the occurrence of neoplasms in several ways through actions in either of the two sequences of carcinogenesis (Figure 1). They could induce neoplastic conversion either by initiating a series of intracellular events leading to DNA alterations, by permanently altering gene expression, or possibly by producing chromosomal alterations. Also, they could enhance the second sequence, neoplastic development through hormonal, immunosuppressive, or promoting effects. In tissues with preexisting neoplastic cells, these latter effects would facilitate the development of neoplasms.

Examples of carcinogens that may indirectly lead to DNA damage include the hypolipidemic drug clofibrate, the plastizer di(2-ethylhexyl)phthalate, and the phorbol ester TPA for which there is evidence that they may generate reactive oxygen species that could lead to DNA damage.[54,55] At high doses, the inorganic chemical hydrazine produces aberrant methylation in DNA,[56] possibly by intracellular formation of a methylating intermediate. These agents are not DNA-reactive as such, and, therefore, differ fundamentally in their properties from carcinogens that are DNA-reactive. Moreover, these agents must produce another biological effect, such as peroxisome proliferation in the case of clofibrate, and cytotoxicity in the case of hydrazine, to create the conditions leading to the generation of the specific moieties suspected to result in genetic damage. Since their action requires an antecedent nongenetic biological effect, such chemicals can appropriately be considered to be epigenetic agents. More evidence is still needed to be certain that DNA damage of the type associated with these agents (e.g., oxidative damage) is essential to their carcinogenicity. If it is, such chemicals eventually may be categorized as indirect genotoxins. In any event, the point must be made that as new evidence on mechanisms of action accumulates, it may turn out that a specific agent or group requires reclassification. This does not mean that the basic distinction is invalid between carcinogens that are primarily and directly DNA-reactive and those that are not.

Perhaps the first modern theory on the basis for the formation of cancer cells was that advanced by Boveri,[57] implicating alteration in chromosomes. The occurrence of chromosomal abnormalities in neoplastic cells is now well-established.[58] Moreover, many carcinogens are known to produce chromosome mutations[35,59,60] DNA aneuploidy and possibly, therefore, chromosome aneuploidy have been reported to occur at early stages of carcinogenesis.[61] If it reasonably can be established that chromosomal alteration in the absence of DNA-reactivity is an event actually leading to neoplastic conversion, then there would be a basis for classifying clastogenic carcinogens as a separate category.

Several types of epigenetic carcinogens have been distinguished (Table 1). These appear to differ in their properties.

A. Neoplasm-Promoting Carcinogens

Neoplasm promotion is defined as the growth augmentation of dormant neoplastic cells,[62] although some use the term to designate any enhancement of carcinogenesis. Neoplasm promotion in the more specific sense could lead to neoplasm development in a tissue that harbors latent neoplastic cells. Such abnormal cells are undoubtedly present in the commonly used inbred laboratory rodents that have a high cryptogenic incidence of certain neoplasms. The cells that give rise to these neoplasms are probably altered by genetic factors, although in some instances, transformation may also be due to exposure to occult environmental carcinogens. Regardless, the tissues in which neoplasms occur certainly contain more preneoplastic cells than that actually develop into neoplasms under normal conditions. Consequently, agents such as phenobarbital and saccharin that promote neoplastic development could increase the incidence of neoplasms in organs that are the site of spontaneous neoplasms by facilitating neoplastic development by cells that otherwise would not be expressed.

Agents that are considered to produce an increase in neoplasia through promoting effects are usually associated with neoplasms in a single organ following long-term administration by themselves; this is the case with phenobarbital and liver neoplasms, saccharin and bladder neoplasms, and butylated hydroxyanisole and forestomach neoplasms; there can also be sharp species differences in effects.[63,64]

Neoplasm promotion can be produced through a variety of mechanisms, including hormone effects and immunosuppression, as will be discussed. An important effect may be inhibition of the communications between cells. Considerable evidence suggests that the proliferation of neoplastic cells can be restrained by their association with normal cells. This could be mediated by transmission to the neoplastic cells of growth and/or differentiation factors from normal cells. If so, interruption of such exchange between cells would serve to release the dormant neoplastic cells from control and permit their development into neoplasms.[65] Inhibition of cell-to-cell communication in cell culture has been demonstrated for a variety of promoters and in several cell systems.[65-72]

Recently, interest has focused on the induction of reactive oxygen species as mediators of promotion.[55] The evidence for this stems almost entirely from studies with TPA and skin carcinogenesis. The fact that antioxidants such as butylated hydroxytoluene and butylated hydroxyanisole are promoters of liver,[73,74] lung,[75] and stomach[76] cancer, respectively, does not support this notion, at least superficially as a general mechanism. Nevertheless, the carcinogenicity of TPA[77] could in part be related to formation of reactive oxygen.

B. Endocrine-Modifying Carcinogens

At unphysiological levels, a variety of hormones has the ability to facilitate neoplasm development in organs whose function they affect.[78] In addition, many chemicals that are not hormonally active can alter the function of endocrine organs, resulting in an abnormal hormonal environment leading to neoplasm development in hormonally responsive tissues. Examples of the latter are amitrole and ethylenethiourea, which affect thyroid function, leading to thyroid hyperplasia and eventually thyroid neoplasms, particularly in rats. Recently, agents that inhibit acid production in the stomach have been found to cause experimental tumors of enterochromaffin-like cells (carcinoids) as a result of prolonged hypergastrinemia stemming from sustained complete achlorhydria in the stomach.[79]

The question of DNA reactivity of steroidal estrogens and the synthetic estrogen diethylstilbestrol is complicated. Metzler[80] has proposed that biotransformation of diethylstilbestrol gives rise to a semiquinone and quinone that could result in DNA damage. Similarly, Liehr[81] has developed evidence supporting the formation of reactive species from estrogens. A few short-term tests have yielded positive results with estrogens and diethylstilbestrol, notably transformation and chromosome assays,[38,60] whereas tests for DNA damage, including in vivo assays,[15a] have been uniformly negative.[21] DNA binding of estrogens has not been found,[17] and diethylstilbestrol showed only very low binding.[82] Thus, the data on DNA-reactivity of estrogens and diethylstilbestrol are largely inconclusive, but most experiments suggest that this is not a significant aspect to their effect on target tissues. Given the fact that these agents produce neoplasms only in hormonally responsive tissues (whereas DNA-reactive carcinogens typically affect tissues where bioactivation is substantial), the overall evidence suggests that estrogenic hormones produce neoplasms through their hormonal effects.

The basis for the carcinogenicity of hormone-modifying agents could be effects in either sequence of carcinogenesis. The stimulation of cell proliferation could enhance neoplastic conversion resulting from spontaneous genetic alterations or the action of occult carcinogens. In addition, certain hormones (particularly estrogen and diethylstilbestrol), either through formation of quinones or alteration of cellular processes, might give rise to reactive oxygen species that could have a DNA-damaging or chromosome-altering effect.

Alternatively, carcinogenesis may result from promotion to tumor formation of preexisting neoplastic cells. Indeed, many hormonal agents have produced an enhancing effect on carcinogenesis when given after a genotoxic carcinogen.[78,83] Regardless of the exact mechanism, modification of the hormonal environment is the main biological effect for these agents, and on this basis they can be distinguished from promoters that do not perturb the endocrine system.

The hormone-modifying carcinogens that affect the thyroid gland exemplify two important features of epigenetic agents: species specificity and reversibility of effects. Amitrole produces thyroid neoplasms in rats, whereas mice and hamsters have been shown not to be susceptible to the thyroid effects.[84] With ethylenethiourea, it has been demonstrated that the thyroid effects are reversible upon cessation of exposure.[85]

C. Immunosuppressant Carcinogens

Many DNA-reactive carcinogens are toxic to cells of the immune system[86] in addition to the other tissues that they affect. This may play some role in their carcinogenicity, but the evidence is not impressive. In addition, there are agents, such as purine analogs, which are not DNA-reactive and whose main site of action is the immune system. Most of these drugs produce primarily lymphomas or leukemias in animals or humans. The discovery that translocation of immunoglobulin genes can be associated with altered expression of oncogenes[87] provides a plausible mechanism whereby agents affecting the immune system could produce neoplastic conversion in cells of this system. Also, by blocking immunological surveillance, immunosuppression could allow escape of suppressed neoplastic cells,[88] thereby affecting the second sequence of carcinogenesis.

D. Cytotoxic Carcinogens

Lethal injury to cells in a tissue could lead to the development of neoplasms through several mechanisms. One means is by stimulating compensatory cell proliferation. This could lead to an increase in the background mutation incidence, as has been proposed for several liver carcinogens of the aliphatic halogenated hydrocarbon type,[12] and may also occur with nitrilotriacetic acid.[89] It is possible that impairment of the fidelity of DNA polymerases could be involved.[90] Increased cell proliferation could also lead to an enhancement of neoplastic conversion produced by occult carcinogens.

Cytotoxicity could also operate in the second sequence of carcinogenesis. In 1938, Haddow[91] proposed that cytotoxic agents could selectively kill normal cells, and thereby permit the survival of preexisting abnormal cells and their development into neoplasms. This concept has been applied to liver carcinogenesis by Tatematsu and co-workers,[92] who have described conditions under which several liver carcinogens injure or kill normal hepatocytes but not altered cells in preneoplastic lesions.

E. Peroxisome-Proliferating Carcinogens

Several structural types of liver carcinogen are now known to increase the numbers of peroxisomes in liver cells.[54] These include hypolipidemic drugs such as clofibrate, fenofibrate, and gemfibrizol, several phthalate esters, and trichloroethylene. The increased peroxisomes have levels of activity of enzymes involved in the β-oxidation of lipids that exceed the elevation of catalase. Consequently, hydrogen peroxide is generated in these peroxisomes and may escape into the cytoplasm, giving rise to reactive hydroxyl radicals. Moreover, some peroxisome proliferators also inhibit the activity of cytoplasmic glutathione peroxidase,[93] which degrades hydrogen peroxide in the cytoplasm. As a result, it seems likely that these agents may give rise to reactive hydroxyl radicals which could damage DNA and lead to neoplastic conversion of hepatocytes. Interestingly, these agents are not effective promoters when given after a genotoxic carcinogen.[94] If the evidence that they give to reactive oxygen species holds up, then the role of such moieties as general mediators of neoplasm promotion[55] becomes further questionable, as discussed earlier.

To summarize the understanding of epigenetic carcinogens, there is substantial and growing evidence that a number of carcinogenic chemicals does not undergo reaction with DNA per se, but rather exerts other cellular effects that seem to be the basis for their carcinogenicity. Such nongenotoxic effects may lead indirectly to genetic alterations resulting in neoplastic conversion, or may facilitate tumor development of dormant neoplastic cells.

The characteristics of the carcinogenicity of epigenetic agents cannot be generalized due to the diversity of modes of action that are involved. Nevertheless, many features differ substantially from those of DNA-reactive carcinogens. In particular, carcinogens of the neoplasm-promoting type have quite distinct characteristics (Table 4). Thus far, very few synthetic carcinogens of the epigenetic type have been linked to human cancer. Of the 23 known human carcinogens listed in Table 3, only 7 (arsenic, asbestos, azathioprine, benzene, conjugated estrogens, diethylstilbestrol, and nickel) are possible epigenetic carcinogens. With most of these, the data base is equivocal, although estrogens and diethylstilbestrol appear to act through a hormonal mechanism, azathioprine through immunosuppression, and asbestos as a solid-state carcinogen. Nevertheless, epigenetic agents are considered to play a major role in the causation of human cancer, primarily as elements to which humans are exposed through voluntary lifestyle practices.[95] A prime example is the association between the consumption of a high fat diet with an increased risk of breast and colon cancer.[96]

IV. CONCLUSIONS

In the past three decades, the understanding of the carcinogenic process has gone

Table 4
CHARACTERISTICS OF CARCINOGENICITY OF NEOPLASM-PROMOTING CARCINOGENS

None demonstrated to be active with single exposure
May be active at low dose, but require a level of exposure to produce relevant biological effect
Additivity uncertain — can inhibit one another
None proven to be active transplacentally
No evidence of enhanced susceptibility of neonates
Shifts in organotropism not reported

through many important evolutions. As discussed in this review, evidence is accruing that carcinogens are not all identical in their mode of action. This understanding has been formalized in the classification proposed by Weisburger and Williams.[15] The present review has not uncovered a single research paper in which evidence was presented to specifically refute this basic distinction between carcinogens that react chemically with DNA and those that produce another biological effect as their primary, critical action. To the contrary, much current research is focusing on actions of carcinogens other than DNA binding.

In evaluating the concept of mechanistically distinct carcinogens, it is important to distinguish between the framework of categorization, and the assignment of specific carcinogens to categories. There will always be uncertainty with specific carcinogens over interpretation of some experiments or tests as to whether the evidence indicates that the chemicals concerned are DNA-reactive or can be characterized by another property. An example discussed here is diethylstilbestrol. Such controversy is the nature of science, and, indeed, the classification of carcinogens was proposed in part to focus on such questions. Nevertheless, even though the properties of one or more specific agents are unresolved, or if new research with an agent shows that it should be reclassified, the basic distinction between carcinogens of different types is not invalidated.

If the concept of mechanistically distinct carcinogens becomes established, it will require researchers to devise more sophisticated means for assessing the potential hazards to humans of specific carcinogens, rather than simply assuming that all agents pose comparable hazards. Clearly, chemicals such as phenobarbital and clofibrate, which must produce biological effects requiring substantial exposures in order to be carcinogenic, differ from bis(chloromethyl)ether and vinyl chloride in their danger to humans. It is undoubtedly for this reason that phenobarbital and clofibrate, although used extensively as human medications, have not been associated with human cancer, in contrast to these DNA-reactive agents.[47] The approaches to hazard assessment which will address such differences seem likely to be based on mechanistic considerations and involve a case-by-case analysis entailing evaluation of all relevant biological effects.[97]

Another important development in cancer research is the recognition that cancer is not one, but many diseases with distinct multifactorial causes. A gradual shift has been taking place from the belief that cancer stems mainly from exposure to a "sea of chemical carcinogens", often presumed to be of industrial origin, to the recognition that some of the most important causative agents in human cancer are voluntary lifestyle practices such as cigarette smoking, heavy alcohol use, and consumption of a diet high in fat and low in fiber in the Western world, or one with excessively salted, pickled, or smoked foods in the Orient and in northern and eastern Europe. Some lifestyle practices result in exposures to DNA-reactive carcinogens, as is the case with pickled or smoked foods and broiled meat.[98] Other practices, such as consumption of a high fat diet, contribute epigenetic enhancing agents.[96] Although practices entailing exposure to either type of agent are associated with an increased risk of cancer, a key difference is that epigenetic effects are reversible up to a point, as discussed for rat thyroid lesions induced by ethylenethiourea. There is also evidence that such effects in humans are reversible; regression of liver tumors has been observed following cessation of use of oral contraceptives,[99] and reduction in risk of endometrial cancer was reported after decrease in estrogen use.[100] In contrast, with exposure to carcinogens of the type now known to be DNA-reactive, risk increases with time.[101] Thus, while efforts must be directed toward identifying both types of agents and minimizing their exposures, a more immediate reduction of disease may be anticipated through control of epigenetic factors. Consequently, the distinction between mechanistically different agents has important public health implications.

REFERENCES

1. Miller, J. A. and Miller, E. C., Chemical carcinogenics: metabolism and approaches to its control, Guest editorial, *J. Natl. Cancer Inst.,* 47, 5, 1971.
2. Magee, P. N., Pegg, A. E., and Swann, P. F., Molecular mechanisms of chemical carcinogenesis, in *Handbuch der allegemeinen Pathologie,* Altman, H. W. et al., Eds., Springer-Verlag, Berlin, 329, 1975.
3. Brookes, P., Role of covalent binding in carcinogenicity, in *Biological Reactive Intermediates Formation, Toxicity and Inactivation,* Jollow, D. J., Kocais, J. J., Snyder, R., and Vainio, H., Eds., Plenum Press, New York, 1977, 470.
4. Malling, H. V., Mutagenicity of two potent carcinogens, dimethylnitrosamine and diethylnitrosamine in *Neurospora crassa, Mutat. Res.,* 3, 537, 1966.
5. Auerbach, C., Robson, J. M., and Carr, J. G., The chemical production of mutations, *Science,* 105, 243, 1947.
6. Ames, B. N., Durston, W. E., Yamasaki, E., and Lee, F. D., Carcinogens are mutagens: a simple test system combining liver homogenates for activation and bacteria for detection, *Proc. Natl. Acad. Sci. U.S.A.,* 70, 2281, 1973.
7. Sugimura, T., Sato, S., Nagao, M., Yahagi, T., Matsushima, T., Seino, Y., Takeuchi, M., and Kawachi, T., in *Fundamental in Cancer Prevention,* Magee, P. N., Takayama, S., Sugimura, T., and Matsushima, T., Eds., University of Tokyo, Tokyo/University Park Press, Baltimore, 1976, 191.
8. Williams, G. M., A comparison of in vivo and in vitro metabolic activation systems, in *Critical Reviews in Toxicology — Strategies for Short-Term Testing for Mutagens/Carcinogens,* Butterworth, B., Ed., CRC Press, Boca Raton, Fla., 1979, 96.
9. Williams, G. M., Review of in vitro test systems using DNA damage and repair for screening of chemical carcinogens, *J. Assoc. Off. Anal. Chem.,* 62, 857, 1979.
10. Kroes, R., Animal data, interpretation and consequences, in *Environmental Carcinogenesis,* Emmelot, P. and Kriek, E., Eds., Elsevier/North-Holland, Amsterdam, 1979, 287.
11. Kolbye, A. C., Impact of short-term screening tests on regulatory action, in *The Predictive Value of Short-Term Screening Tests in Carcinogenicity Evaluation,* Williams, G. M., Kroes, R., Waaijers, H. W., and van de Poll, K. W., Eds., Elsevier/North-Holland, Amsterdam, 1980, 311.
12. Stott, W. T., Reitz, R. H., Schumann, A. M., and Watanabe, P. G., Genetic and nongenetic events in neoplasia, *Food Cosmet. Toxicol.,* 19, 567, 1981.
13. Truhaut, R., Some comments on the advantages and limitations of short-term tests for the evaluation of the carcinogenic potentiabilities of chemicals, in *Short-Term Tests for Carcinogenesis,* Garrattini, S., Mazue, G., Roncucci, R., and Williams, G. M., Eds., Elsevier, Amsterdam, 1983, 342.
14. Miller, E. C. and Miller, J. A., Milestones in chemical carcinogenesis, *Semin. Oncol.,* 6, 445, 1979.
15. Weisburger, J. H. and Williams, G. M., Chemical carcinogens, in *Toxicology. The Basic Science of Poisons,* 2nd ed., Doull, J., Classen, C. D., and Amdur, M. O., Eds., Macmillan, New York, 84, 1980.
15a. Yager, J. D., Jr. and Fifield, D. S., Jr., Lack of hepatogenotoxicity of oral contraceptive steroids, *Carcinogenesis,* 3, 625, 1982.
16. Reddy, M. V., Gupta, R. C., Randerath, E., and Randerath, K., 32p-Postlabeling test for covalent DNA binding of chemicals *in vivo:* application to a variety of aromatic carcinogens and methylating agents, *Carcinogenesis,* 5, 231, 1984.

17. Caviezel, M., Lutz, W. K., Minini, U., and Schlatter, C., Interaction of estrone and estradiol with DNA and protein of liver and kidney in rat and hamster in vivo and in vitro, *Arch. Toxicol.,* 55, 97, 1984.
18. Pienta, R. J., Kushner, L. M., and Russell, L. S., The use of short-term tests and limited bioassays in carcinogenicity testing, *Reg. Toxicol. Pharmacol.,* 4, 249, 1984.
19. Turnbull, D. and Rodricks, J. V., Assessment of possible carcinogenic risk to humans resulting from exposure to di(2-ethylhexyl)phthalate (DEHP), *J. Am. Coll. Toxicol.,* 4, 111, 1985.
20. International Agency for Research on Cancer, Approaches to Classifying Chemical Carcinogens According to Mechanism of Action, Internal Tech. Rep. No. 83/001, IARC, Lyon, 1983.
21. Upton, A. C., Clayson, D. G., Jansen, J. D., Rosenkranz, H., and Williams, G. M., Report of ICPEMC task group on the differentiation between genotoxic and nongenotoxic carcinogens, *Mutat. Res.,* 133, 1, 1984.
22. Office of Science and Technology Policy, Chemical Carcinogens; a Review of the Science and its Associated Principles, Part II, Fed. Regist., 50, 10372, 1985.
23. Weinstein, I. B., Carcinogen policy at EPA, *Science,* 219, 794, 1983.
24. Lijinsky, W., Carcinogenic risk. Letter, *Science,* 221, 810, 1983.
25. Montessano, R. and Slaga, T. J., Initiation and promotion in carcinogenesis: an appraisal, *Cancer Surv.,* 2, 613, 1983.
26. Harper, B. L. and Morris, D. L., Implications of multiple mechanisms of carcinogenesis for short-term testing, *Teratogen. Carcinogen. Mutagen.,* 4, 483, 1984.
27. Perera, F. P., The genotoxic/epigenetic distinction: relevance to cancer policy, *Environ. Res.,* 34, 175, 1985.
28. Ehrenberg, L., Brookes, P., Druckrey, H., Lagerlof, B., Litwin, J., and Williams, G. M., The relation of cancer induction and genetic damage, in *Evaluation of Genetic Risks of Environmental Chemicals,* Ramel, C., Ed., Ambio Special Report No. 3, Royal Swedish Academy of Sciences, Universitetsforlaget, Stockholm, 15, 1973.
29. **Williams, G. M. and Weisburger, J. H.,** Chemical carcinogens, in *Toxicology — The Basic Sciences of Poisons,* 3rd ed., Klassen, C., Amdur, M., and Doull, J., Eds., Macmillan, New York, 1986, 99.
30. Lutz, W. K., In vivo covalent binding of organic chemicals to DNA as a quantitative indicator in the process of chemical carcinogenesis, *Mutat. Res.,* 65, 289, 1979.
31. Poirier, M. C., Antibodies to carcinogen-DNA adducts, *J. Natl. Cancer Inst.,* 67, 515, 1981.
32. Osborne, M. R., DNA interactions of reactive intermediates derived from carcinogens, in *Chemical Carcinogens,* 2nd ed., Searle, C. E., Ed., American Chemical Society, Washington, D.C., 1984, 485.
33. Weisburger, J. H. and Williams, G. M., Carcinogen testing, current problems and new approaches, *Science,* 214, 401, 1981.
34. Williams, G. M., Indices for identification of genotoxic and epigenetic carcinogens in cell culture, in *Application of Biological Markers to Carcinogen Testing,* Milman, H. A. and Sell, S., Eds., Plenum Press, New York, 1983, 165.
35. **Ishidate, M., Jr., Sofuni, T., and Yoshikawa, K.,** Chromosomal aberration tests in vitro as a primary screening tool for environmental mutagens and/or carcinogens, *Gann Monogr. Cancer Res.,* 27, 95, 1981.
36. Tsutsui, T., Maizumi, H., and Barrett, J. C., Colcemid-induced plastic transformation and aneuploidy in Syrian hamster embryo cells, *Carcinogenesis,* 5, 89, 1984.
37. IARC/NCI/EPA Working Group, Cellular and molecular mechanisms of cell transformation and standardization of transformation assays of established cell lines for the prediction of carcinogenic chemicals: overview and recommended protocols, *Cancer Res.,* 45, 2395, 1985.
38. Pienta, R. J., Evaluation and relevance of the Syrian hamster embryo cell system, in *Predictive Value of Short-Term Screening Tests in Carcinogenicity Evaluation,* Williams, G. M., Kroes, R., Waaijers, H. W., and van de Poll, K. W., Eds., *(Appl. Meth. Oncol. Ser.,* Vol. 3), Elsevier, New York, 1980, 149.
39. Evans, H. J., Cytogenic methods for detecting effects of chemical mutagens, *Ann. N.Y. Acad. Sci.,* 407, 131, 1983.
40. Bradley, M. O., Chang Hsu, Ih., and Harris, C. C., Relationship between sister chromatoid exchange and mutagenicity, toxicity and DNA damage, *Nature (London),* 282, 318, 1979.
41. Carrano, A. V. and Thompson, L. H., Sister chromatid exchange and gene mutation, *Cytogenet. Cell Genet.,* 33, 57, 1982.
42. Emerit, I., Levy, A., and Cerutti, P. A., Suppression of tumor promoter phorbol 12-myristate acetate-induced chromosome breakage by antioxidants and inhibitors of arachidonic acid metabolism, *Mutat. Res.,* 110, 327, 1983.
43. Weisburger, J. H. and Williams, G. M., Metabolism of chemical carcinogens, in *Cancer: A Comprehensive Treatise,* 2nd ed., Becker, F., Ed., Plenum Press, New York, 1982, 241.

44. Cooper, G. M., Cellular transforming genes, *Science*, 218, 801, 1982.
45. Land, H., Parada, L. F., and Weinberg, R. A., Cellular oncogenes and multistep carcinogenesis, *Science*, 222, 771, 1983.
46. Bishop, J. M., Viral oncogenes, *Cell*, 42, 23, 1985.
47. International Agency for Research on Cancer, Monographs on the Evaluation of the Carcinogenic Risk of Chemicals to Humans, Chemicals, Industrial Processes and Industries Associated with Cancer in Humans, Vol. 1 to 29, Suppl. 4, IARC, Lyon, 1982.
48. Lutz, W. K. and Schlatter, C., Saccharin does not bind to DNA of liver or bladder in the rat, *Chem. Biol. Interact.*, 19, 253, 1977.
49. Diaz Gomez, M. I. and Castro, J. A., Convalent binding of chloroform metabolites to nuclear proteins — no evidence for binding of nucleic acids, *Cancer Lett.*, 9, 213, 1980.
50. Schumann, A. M., Quast, J. F., and Wantanabe, P. G., The pharmacokinetics and macromolecular interactions of perchloroethylene in mice and rat as related to oncogenicity, *Toxicol. Appl. Pharmacol.*, 55, 207, 1980.
51. Laib, R. J., Stockle, G., Bolt, H. M., and Kunz, W., Vinyl chloride and trichloroethylene: comparison of alkylating effects of metabolites and induction of preneoplastic enzyme deficiencies in rat liver, *J. Cancer Res. Clin. Oncol.*, 94, 139, 1979.
52. Parchman, L. G. and Magee, P. N., Metabolism of [^{14}C] trichloroethylene to $^{14}CO_2$ and interaction of a metabolite with liver DNA in rats and mice, *J. Toxicol. Environ. Health*, 9, 797, 1982.
53. Von Daniken, A., Lutz, W. K., Jackh, R., and Schlatter, C., Investigation of the potential for binding of di(2-ethylhexyl)phthalate (DEHP) and di(2-ethylhexyl)adipate (DEHA) to liver DNA in vivo, *Toxicol. Appl. Pharmacol.*, 73, 373, 1984.
54. Reddy, J. K. and Lalwani, N. D., Carcinogenesis by hepatic peroxisome proliferators: evaluation of the risk of hypolipidemic drugs and industrial plasticizers to humans, *Crit. Rev. Toxicol.*, 12, 1, 1983.
55. Troll, W. and Wiesner, R., The role of oxygen radicals as a possible mechanism of tumor promotion, *Annu. Rev. Pharmacol. Toxicol.*, 25, 509, 1985.
56. Bosan, W. S. and Shank, R. C., Methylation of liver DNA guanine in hamsters given hydrazine, *Toxicol. Appl. Pharmacol.*, 70, 324, 1983.
57. Boveri, T., *The Origin of Malignant Tumors*, Williams & Wilkins, Baltimore, 1929.
58. Yunis, J. J., The chromosomal basis of human neoplasia, *Science*, 221, 227, 1983.
59. Preston, R. J., Au, W., Bender, M. A., Brewer, J. G., Carrano, A. V., Heddle, J. A., McFee, A. F., Wolff, S., and Wassom, J. S., Mammalian in vivo and in vitro cytogenetic assays: a report of the U.S. EPA's Gene-Tox program, *Mutat. Res.*, 87, 143, 1981.
60. Tsutsui, T., Maisumi, H., McLachlan, J. A., and Barrett, J. C., Aneuploidy induction and cell transformation by diethylstilbestrol: a possible chromosomal mechanism in carcinogenesis, *Cancer Res.*, 43, 3814, 1983.
61. Mori, H., Tanaka, T., Sugie, S., Takahashi, M., and Williams, G. M., DNA content of liver cell nuclei of N-2-fluorenyl acetamide induced altered foci and neoplasms in rats and human hyperplastic foci, *J. Natl. Cancer Inst.*, 69, 1277, 1982.
62. Berenblum, I., *Carcinogenesis as a Biological Problem*, Vol. 34, North-Holland, Amsterdam, 1974.
63. Fukushima, S., Arai, M., Nakanowatari, J., Hikino, T., Okuda, M., and Ito, N., Differences in susceptibility to sodium saccharin among various strains of rats and other animal species, *Gann*, 74, 8, 1983.
64. Stenback, F., Mori, H., Furuya, K., and Williams, G. M., The pathogenesis of dimethylnitrosamine-induced hepatocellular cancer in hamster liver and a lack of enhancement by phenobarbital, *J. Natl. Cancer Inst.*, 76, 327, 1986.
65. Williams, G. M., Liver carcinogenesis: the role for some chemicals of an epigenetic mechanism of liver tumor promotion involving modification of the cell membrane, *Food Cosmet. Toxicol.*, 19, 577, 1981.
66. Yotti, L. P., Chang, C. C., and Trosko, J. E., Elimination of metabolic cooperation in Chinese hamster cells by a tumour promoter, *Science*, 206, 1089, 1979.
67. Murray, A. W. and Fitzgerald, D. J., Tumor promoters inhibit metabolic cooperation in cocultures of epidermal and 3T3 cells, *Biochem. Biophys. Res. Commun.*, 91, 395, 1979.
68. Trosko, J. E., Yotti, L. P., Dawson, B., and Chang, C. C., In vitro assay for tumor promoters, in *Short-Term Tests for Chemical Carcinogens*, Stich, H. F. and San, R. H. C., Eds., Springer-Verlag, New York, 1981, 420.
69. Williams, G. M., Telang, S., and Tong, C., Inhibition of intercellular communication between liver cells by the liver tumor promoter 1,1,1-trichloro-2,2-bis (P-chlorophenyl) ethane (DDT), *Cancer Lett.*, 11, 339, 1981.
70. Noda, K., Umeda, M., and Ono, T., Effects of various chemicals including bile acids and chemical carcinogens on the inhibition of metabolic cooperation, *Gann*, 72, 772, 1981.

71. Newbold, R. F. and Amos, J., Inhibition of metabolic cooperation between mammalian cells in culture by tumour promoters, *Carcinogenesis*, 2, 243, 1981.

72. Jone, C. M., Trosko, J. E., Chang, C. C., Fujiki, H., and Sugimura, T., Inhibition of intercellular communication in Chinese hamster V79 cells by teleocidin, *Gann*, 73, 874, 1982.

73. Peraino, C., Fry, R. J. M., Staffeldt, E., and Christopher, J. P., Enhancing effects of phenobarbitone and butylated hydroxytoluene on 2-acetylaminofluorene-induced hepatotumorigenesis in the rat, *Food Cosmet. Toxicol.*, 15, 93, 1977.

74. Maeura, Y. and Williams, G. M., Enhancing effect of butylated hydroxytoluene on the development of liver altered foci and neoplasms induced by N-2-fluorenylacetamide in rats, *Food Cosmet. Toxicol.*, 22, 191, 1984.

75. Witchi, H. P., Enhancement of tumor formation in mouse lung by dietary butylated hydroxytoluene, *Toxicology*, 21, 95, 1981.

76. Imaida, K., Fukushima, S., Shirai, T., Masui, T., Ogiso, T., and Ito, N., Promoting activities of butylated hydroxyanisole, butylated hydroxytoluene and sodium L-ascorbate on forestomach and urinary bladder carcinogenesis initiated with methylnitrosourea in F344 male rats, *Gann*, 75, 769, 1984.

77. Iversen, U. M. and Iversen, O. H., The carcinogenic effect of TPA (12-O-tetradecanoylphorbol-13-acetate) when applied to the skin of hairless mice, *Virchows Arch. B*, 30, 33, 1979.

78. Furth, J., Hormones as etiological agents in neoplasia, in *Cancer, A Comprehensive Treatise*, Becker, F. F., Ed., Plenum Press, New York, 1982, 89.

79. Ekman, L., Hansson, E., Havu, N., Carlsson, E., and Lundberg, C., Toxicological studies on omeprazole, *Scand. J. Gastroenterol.*, 20(Suppl. 108), 53, 1985.

80. Metzler, M., Metabolism of stilbene estrogens and steroidal estrogens in relation to carcinogenicity, *Arch. Toxicol.*, 55, 104, 1984.

81. Liehr, J. C., Modulation of estrogen-induced carcinogenesis by chemical modifications, *Arch. Toxicol.*, 55, 119, 1984.

82. Lutz, W. K., Jaggi, W., and Schlatter, C., Covalent binding of diethylstilbestral to DNA in rat and hamster liver and kidney, *Chem. Biol. Interact.*, 42, 251, 1982.

83. Yager, J. E., Campbell, H. A., Longnecker, D. S., Roebuck, B. D., and Benoit, M. C., Enhancement of hepatocarcinogenesis in female rats by ethinyl estradiol and mestranol but not estradiol, *Cancer Res.*, 44, 3862, 1984.

84. Steinhoff, D., Webber, H., Mohr, U., and Boehme, K., Evaluation of amitrole (aminotriazole) for potential carcinogenicity in orally dosed rats, mice, and golden hamsters, *Toxicol. Appl. Pharmacol.*, 69, 161, 1983.

85. Arnold, D. L., Krewski, D. R., Junkins, D. B., McGuire, P. F., Moodie, C. A., and Munro, I. C., Reversibility of ethylenethiourea-induced thyroid lesions, *Toxicol. Appl. Pharmacol.*, 67, 264, 1983.

86. Melief, C. T. M. and Schwartz, R. S., Immunocompetence and malignancy, in *Cancer, A Comprehensive Treatise*, Vol. 1, 2nd ed., Becker, F. F., Ed., Plenum Press, New York, 1982, 161.

87. Leder, P., Battey, J., Lenoir, G., Moulding, C., Murphy, W., Potter, H., Stewart, T., and Taub, R., Translocations among antibody genes in human cancer, *Science*, 222, 765, 1983.

88. Burnet, F. M., The concept of immunological surveillance, *Prog. Exp. Tumor Res.*, 13, 1, 1970.

89. Anderson, R. L., Bishop, W. E., and Campbell, R. L., A review of the environmental and mammalian toxicology of nitrolotriacetic acid, *Crit. Rev. Toxicol.*, 15, 1, 1985.

90. Sirover, M. A. and Loeb, L. A., On the fidelity of DNA synthesis: effects of steroids and intercalating agents, *Chem. Biol. Interact.*, 30, 1, 1980.

91. Haddow, A., Cellular inhibition and the origin of cancer, *Acta Unio Int. Contra Cancrum*, 3, 342, 1938.

92. Tatematsu, M., Kaku, T., Medline, A., Eriksson, L., Roomi, W., Sharma, R. N., Murray, R. K., and Farber, E., Markers of liver neoplasia — real or fictional?, in *Application of Biological Markers to Carcinogen Testing*, Milman, H. A. and Sell, S. E., Eds., Plenum Press, New York, 1983, 25.

93. Furukawa, K., Numoto, S., Furuya, K., Furukawa, N., and Williams, G. M., Effect of the hepatocarcinogen nafenopin, a peroxisome proliferator, on the activities of rat liver glutathione requiring enzymes and catalase in comparison to the action of phenobarbital, *Cancer Res.*, 45, 5011, 1985.

94. Numoto, S., Furukawa, K., Furuya, K., and Williams, G. M., Effects of the hepatocarcinogenic peroxisome-proliferating agents clofibrate and nafenopin on the rat liver cell membrane enzymes glutamyltranspeptidase and alkaline phosphatase and on the early stages of liver carcinogenesis, *Carcinogenesis*, 5, 1603, 1984.

95. Weisburger, J. H. and Williams, G. M., Chemical carcinogenesis, in *Cancer Medicine*, Holland, J. F. and Frei, E., III, Lea & Febiger, Philadelphia, 1982, 42.

96. Reddy, B. S., Cohen, L. A., McCoy, G. D., Hill, P., Weisburger, J. H., and Wynder, E. L., Nutrition and its relationship to cancer, *Adv. Cancer Res.*, 32, 237, 1980.

97. Grice, H. C., Ed., Interpretation and extrapolation of chemical and biological carcinogenicity data to establish human safety standards, in *Current Issues in Toxicology*, Springer-Verlag, New York, 1984, 1.

98. Sugimura, T. and Sato, S., Mutagens-carcinogens in foods, *Cancer Res.*, Suppl. 43, 2415, 1983.

99. Buhler, H., Pirouino, M., Akovbiantz, A., Altorfer, J., Weitzel, M., Maranta, E., and Schmid, M., Regression of liver cell adenoma, a follow-up study of three consecutive patients after discontinuation of oral contraceptive use, *Gastroenterology*, 82, 775, 1982.

100. Austin, D. F. and Roe, K. M., The decreasing incidence of endometrial cancer: public health implications, *Am. J. Publ. Health*, 72, 65, 1982.

101. Druckrey, H., Quantitative aspects in chemical carcinogenesis, in *Potential Carcinogenic Hazards from Drugs*, UICC Monogr. Ser. Vol. 7, Truhaut, R., Ed., Springer-Verlag, Berlin, 1967, 60.

Chapter 8

RELATIONSHIP BETWEEN MUTAGENESIS AND CARCINOGENESIS

J. Carl Barrett

TABLE OF CONTENTS

I. INTRODUCTION

The correlation between chemically induced mutagenesis and carcinogenesis is one of the key lines of evidence supporting the somatic mutation theory of carcinogenesis, and is a major theoretical justification for using mutagenesis tests to identify potentially carcinogenic chemicals (see Chapter 1). The pioneering work of the Millers[2] demonstrated that many potent carcinogens were not active in the parent form, but had to be metabolically activated to electrophilic intermediates, the ultimate carcinogenic species, which are DNA-reactive, mutagenic, and carcinogenic. With the development of mutagenesis assays and metabolic activation systems, Ames and co-workers[3,4] were able to demonstrate a high degree (~90%) of correlation between mutagenicity and carcinogenicity of chemicals. However, one of the problems in understanding the relationship between these two processes has been the existence of chemicals which appear to be exceptions to this correlation, i.e., mutagens which are not carcinogens, or carcinogens which are not mutagens.[1] In this chapter, I would like to discuss some of these exceptions in order to illustrate the complexity of the carcinogenic problem and to demonstrate that both genetic and epigenetic mechanisms are involved in cancer development.

II. HORMONAL CARCINOGENESIS

The ability of nonmutagenic hormones to induce and/or promote carcinogenesis in a number of species and organs has been cited as evidence for an epigenetic basis of carcinogenesis.[5,6] The natural estrogen 17β-estradiol increases the incidences of mammary, pituitary, uterine, cervical, vaginal, and lymphoid tumors, and interstitial-cell tumors of the testes in mice; it also increases the incidences of mammary and pituitary tumors in rats and renal tumors in hamsters.[6] Similarly, the synthetic estrogen diethylstilbestrol (DES) increases the incidences of mammary tumors, lymphoid tumors, interstitial-cell tumors of the testes, cervical tumors, and vaginal tumors in mice; pituitary, mammary, and bladder tumors in rats; and renal tumors in hamsters.[6] It has been proposed that estrogens are carcinogenic due to their ability to stimulate cell proliferation.[5,7] This hypothesis is supported by experimental observations of tumor-promoting effects of estrogens on carcinogen-initiated mammary cancers,[8,9] hepatocarcinogenesis,[10,11] and vaginal tumors.[12] Analyses of the influence of hormonal factors on human breast cancers also indicate an effect on a late stage in the carcinogenesis process, consistent with a promotional effect.[13,14] Therefore, there is strong evidence from several systems in support of the hypothesis that estrogens are epigenetic carcinogens acting via a promoting effect related to cellular proliferation. The hormonal dependence of transplantable tumors is also in agreement with this proposed mechanism of action.[15]

Despite the convincing evidence that estrogens have an epigenetic effect on carcinogenesis, there are observations which indicate that estrogens induce heritable alterations important in neoplastic development. DES can induce tumors in humans and experimental animals following single or short-term prenatal exposure.[6,16-21] The offspring of treated animals have increased tumor incidences even though not exposed to further treatment. Thus, DES induces a heritable predisposition for certain tumors. In this manner, it resembles tumor initiators,[22] although its mechanism of action may be quite different. Prenatal exposure to DES also induces irreversible changes in differentiation of the cervicovaginal epithelium.[16-18,20,21] Thus, DES "initiation" may arise by a heritable, epigenetic mechanism.

However, there is also evidence that the estrogenic activity is not sufficient to explain the carcinogenic activity of estrogens in certain target tissues. DES can induce preneo-plastic alterations in growth and morphology of diploid cells in culture; the ability of DES-related chemicals to induce cell transformation does not correlate with their estrogenic properties.[23] In the hamster kidney model, renal tumors are induced in vivo by a variety of estrogens, and the tumors which form are estrogen-dependent,[24] indicating an important epigenetic mechanism in the genesis and maintenance of this tumor. However, not all estrogens are active in inducing this tumor. Tumors are induced equally well by DES and 17β-estradiol, but ethinyl estradiol has only weak carcinogenic activity even though it competes equally well with DES and 17β-estradiol for estrogen receptors and has activity similar to carcinogenic estrogens in inducing renal progesterone receptor and serum prolactin levels.[25] Similarly, 2-fluoroestradiol does not induce renal clear-cell carcinomas in hamsters despite its estrogenic potency.[25] One hypothesis to explain the weak carcinogenicity of ethinyl estradiol and 2-fluoroestradiol is that they are poor substrates for catechol estrogen formation.[26-28] A better correlation with carcinogenic activity is observed with metabolism to catechol estrogen than with estrogenic activity in this tumor model.[23,26-29] Also, catechol estrogen formation is greater in kidneys of animals susceptible to the carcinogenic activity of estrogens;[27] agents which inhibit catechol formation in the kidney such as α-naphthoflavone and ascorbic acid inhibit estrogen-induced renal tumors.[27,30] Taken together, these data support the hypothesis that metabolism of estrogens plays a role in their carcinogenic activity, analogous to the metabolic activation requirement for other chemical carcinogens.[30,31] This hypothesis also explains certain observations on estrogen-induced hepatocellular carcinoma in Syrian hamsters. Synthetic estrogens only induce these tumors when the animals are treated with α-naphthoflavone, which alters the metabolism of estrogens in this tissue.[32] Thus, in addition to effects on cell proliferation in estrogen-dependent tissues, estrogens may have the ability to induce heritable alterations in cells. The latter may result from reactive intermediates following metabolic activation.[33,34] Further support for a mutational activity of hormones is provided from in vitro studies.

DES and 17β-estradiol have been reported to be inactive in several mutational assays with bacteria[34-36] and mammalian cells.[37-40] However, there are some reports which indicate genotoxic effects of DES in certain test systems, which seem to conflict with the negative findings cited earlier. DES is mutagenic in mouse lymphoma cells in the presence of a rat liver postmitochondrial supernatant.[41,42] Martin et al.[43] reported that DES induces unscheduled DNA synthesis (UDS) in HeLa cells treated in the presence of rat liver homogenate, while Althaus et al.[44] found no effect of DES on UDS in cultured rat hepatocytes. Rudiger et al.[36] reported that DES and some of its metabolites induce sister-chromatid exchanges in human fibroblasts in culture. Hill and Wolff[45] observed that DES induces sister-chromatic exchanges in lymphocytes from pregnant and premenopausal women, but had only a small effect on lymphocytes from men and postmenopausal women. On the other hand, Abe and Sasaki[46] failed to observe an effect of DES on sister-chromatid exchanges in Chinese hamster cells.

Tsutsui et al.[47] have proposed that those seemingly conflicting results can be explained on the basis of the metabolic activation systems used in the study. These authors have shown that UDS induction in Syrian hamster embryo cells, which have some endogenous metabolizing activity for DES,[48] depends on an exogenous metabolizing system. Under these conditions, qualitative and quantitative differences in the metabolism of DES occur, resulting in a generation of DNA-damaging and mutagenic species.[47] These results are possibly consistent with the in vivo results in the hamster kidney and liver discussed earlier.[24-27] Liehr et al.[49] have recently reported the detection of covalent DES-induced adducts in the DNA of hamster kidneys preceding DES-induced tumors in this organ. These adducts were target organ-specific, but occurred at a very low level. This possibly represents evidence for tumor initiation by DES via damage to cellular macromolecules.[49] Based on the entirety of the results available to date, one has to conclude that DES has some mutagenic activity depending on metabolic activation, and this may be important in its target organ-specific carcinogenic action.[29,31,49]

In addition to the DNA-damaging and mutagenic activity described earlier, DES as well as 17β-estradiol can induce genetic changes by another mechanism not involving direct DNA interaction. Several groups have recently shown that DES binds with microtubules and disrupts tubulin assembly in vivo and in vitro.[50-52] Estrogens, including DES and 17β-estradiol, can cause mitotic abnormalities and numerical chromosome changes in a variety of cells.[5,53-65] The interaction with microtubules provides a biochemical mechanism for the aneuploidy-inducing effects of estrogens.[64]

The possible importance of aneuploidy induction in hormonal carcinogenesis is suggested from cell-transformation studies. DES has been shown to induce morphological and neoplastic transformation of normal, diploid Syrian hamster embryo cells in culture.[38,66] Transformation is induced in the absence of measurable gene mutations[38] or DNA damage.[47] However, treatment of the cells with DES does result in induction of numerical chromosome changes, which has the same cell-cycle dependence and dose-response curve as the induction of cell transformation.[63] Chromosome analysis of the transformed cells also indicates that aneuploidy is a key event in this process.[5,64] The aneuploid nature of in vivo dysplasias studied in DES-exposed females is also consistent with this mechanism, playing a role in the development of human tumors.[67]

In conclusion, it is clear that hormones effect carcinogenesis by epigenetic mechanisms such as stimulation of cell proliferation of estrogen-dependent target cells; in addition, significant evidence exists that certain estrogens can also cause genetic alterations by different mechanisms. These findings indicate that hormonal carcinogenesis is most likely a result of the interplay of genetic and epigenetic factors.

III. FOREIGN BODY, ASBESTOS, AND MINERAL FIBER CARCINOGENESIS

Inert foreign bodies, such as plastic disks and other nonbiodegradable materials, are carcinogenic when implanted subcutaneously in mice.[68] These insults are cited as examples of nonmutagenic carcinogens because no clear demonstration of a genetic mechanism by which they may exert their activity has been demonstrated. The physical properties of these substances are important in their tumorigenic potential. Plastic disks of a certain size are carcinogenic in mice, and this potential is destroyed if the disks are ground and injected as a pulverized powder or if holes are punched into the disks.[68] These experiments indicate that the carcinogenicity is not caused by contaminating chemicals, which should be released and still active following these treatments. Asbestos and other mineral fibers are also carcinogenic in animals and man, and similarities exist between foreign body carcinogenesis and asbestos carcinogenesis.[68] In terms of induction of mesotheliomas in rats following intrapleural injection, the physical rather than the chemical nature of the fibers is related to the carcinogenic potential of diverse mineral dusts.[69] For example, long (>8 μm) and thin (<.25 μm) fibers are more active in mesothelioma induction in rats than short, thick fibers, regardless of the chemical nature of the fibers.[69] Asbestos and other fibers are also cited as examples of nonmutagenic carcinogens.[70]

It has been proposed that asbestos carcinogenicity is the result of its cocarcinogenic and/or tumor-promoting activity.[71-75] This hypothesis is based on the lack of mutagenicity of mineral fibers, the synergism between fibers and carcinogens and smoking, the ability of fibers to cause hyperplasia and metaplasia, and the effects of fibers on cel-

effects on gene expression (see Chapter 1), but defines the action of the chemical; this can create considerable confusion. For example, a chemical (e.g., oxygen radicals or spindle poisons) which does not react directly with DNA, but results by an indirect mechanism in a genetic change such as a chromosome rearrangement or aneuploidy, would be called an epigenetic carcinogen by William's terminology. It is a nonsequitur to call a chemical which induces a genetic change an epigenetic chemical. The emphasis is changed from describing the phenotype of the cell to the mechanism of the chemical. Likewise, DNA-reactive chemicals (for example methylating agents) may cause heritable, epigenetic cellular changes by altering DNA methylation (see Chapter 2) or gene expression.[130] Should these chemicals be called genotoxic or epigenetic? According to William's classification, they are genotoxic, while their mechanism of action involves an epigenetic change.

The need to understand the mechanism(s) of chemical carcinogens is clearly evident. However, the exercise of classifying chemicals according to mechanism has certain inherent difficulties. It was concluded by a working group of the International Agency for Research on Cancer that no classification of chemicals according to mechanisms could be exhaustive or definitive.[132]

In addition, many chemical carcinogens operate via a combination of mechanisms, and even their primary mechanism of action may vary depending on the target cells. For example, some chemicals are complete carcinogens in one tissue, promoters in another, and initiators in another. Classification of chemicals into a single category may be misleading and hinder our comprehensive understanding of the complex problem of chemical carcinogens.

One possible advantage of classification of certain chemicals is to distinguish chemicals with different dose-response characteristics, in particular chemicals for which a threshold exists. This is an area about which too little is currently known to make any conclusions. It is this author's opinion that chemicals exhibiting a threshold dose-response will be identified, but this response will be related to the individual characteristics of a given chemical and not to its characteristic biological activity. Both mutagenic and nonmutagenic chemicals may exhibit thresholds, and likewise chemicals may exert epigenetic effects with a linear dose-response. Therefore, no generalizations can be made, and each chemical will require independent analysis.

VIII. CONCLUSION

Carcinogenesis is a multistep, multigenic, multicausal process (see Chapters 9 through 13, Volume II). As such, both epigenetic and genetic factors are probably important. Thus, it should not be surprising that chemicals which are carcinogenic often have the ability to induce both types of changes. Even carcinogenic insults originally believed to be nonmutagenic, such as hormones, foreign bodies, and asbestos fibers, have been shown to have genetic activities. In part this has been due to the recognition that chromosomal mutations are important in carcinogenesis and that some carcinogens can induce chromosomal mutations without inducing gene mutations. However, tumor-promoting effects, possibly via epigenetic mechanisms, may also be part of the carcinogenic activity of these chemicals. These mechanisms are not mutually exclusive; rather they probably work in conjunction to result in neoplastic progression.

REFERENCES

1. Barrett, J. C., Genetic and epigenetic mechanisms of carcinogenesis, in *Mechanisms of Envrionmental Carcinogenesis,* Vol. 1, Barrett, J. C., Ed., CRC Press, Boca Raton, Fla., 1987, chap. 1.
2. Miller, E. C. and Miller, J. A., The mutagenicity of chemical carcinogens: correlations, problems and interpretations, in *Chemical Mutagenesis,* Vol. 1, Hollaender, A., Ed., Plenum Press, New York, 1971, 83.
3. McCann, J. and Ames, B. N., Detection of carcinogens as mutagens in the Salmonella/microsome test: assay of 300 chemicals. Discussion, *Proc. Natl. Acad. Sci. U.S.A.,* 73, 950, 1976.
4. Ames, B. N., Durston, W. E., Yamasaki, E., and Lee, F. D., Carcinogens are mutagens: a simple test system combining liver homogenates for activation and bacteria for detection, *Proc. Natl. Acad. Sci. U.S.A.,* 70, 2281, 1973.
5. Barrett, J. C., Hesterberg, T. W., Oshimura, M., and Tsutsui, T., Role of chemically induced mutagenic events in neoplastic transformation of Syrian hamster embryo cells, in *Carcinogenesis: A Comprehensive Survey,* Vol. 9, Barrett, J. C. and Tennant, R. W., Eds., Raven Press, New York, 1985, 123.
6. International Agency for Research on Cancer, *Evaluation of Carcinogenic Risk of Chemicals to Humans, Sex Hormones* (II), Vol. 21, IARC, Lyon, 1979.
7. Nandi, S., Role of hormones in mammary neoplasia, *Cancer Res.,* 38, 4046, 1978.
8. Grubbs, C. J., Peckham, J. C., and McDonough, K. D., Effects of ovarian hormones on the induction of 1-methyl-1-nitrosourea-induced mammary cancer, *Carcinogenesis,* 4, 495, 1983.
9. Noronha, R. F. X. and Goodall, C. M., The effects of estrogen on single dose dimethylnitrosamine carcinogenesis in male inbred Crl/CDF rats, *Carcinogenesis,* 5, 1003, 1984.
10. Yager, J. D., Jr. and Yager, R., Oral contraceptive steroids as promoters of hepatocarcinogenesis in female Sprague-Dawley rats, *Cancer Res.,* 40, 3680, 1980.
11. Yager, J. D., Campbell, H. A., Longneck, D. S., Roebuck, B. D., and Benoit, M. C., Enhancement of hepatocarcinogenesis in female rats by ethinyl estradiol and mestranol but not estradiol, *Cancer Res.,* 44, 3862, 1984.
12. Sheehan, D. M., Frederick, C. B., Branham, S., and Heath, J. E., Evidence for estradiol promotion of neoplastic lesions in the rat vagina after initiation with N-methyl-N-nitrosourea, *Carcinogenesis,* 3, 957, 1982.
13. Kaldor, J. M. and Day, N. E., Interpretation of epidemiological studies on the context of the multistage model of carcinogenesis, in *Mechanisms of Environmental Carcinogenesis,* Vol. 2, Barrett, J. C., Ed., CRC Press, Boca Raton, Fla., 1987, chap. 10.
14. Moolgavkar, S. H. and Knudson, A. G., Mutation and cancer: a model for human carcinogenesis, *J. Natl. Cancer Inst.,* 66, 1037, 1981.
15. Satyaswaroop, P. G., Zaino, R. J., and Mortel, R., Human endometrial adenocarcinoma transplanted into nude mice: growth regulation by estradiol, *Science,* 219, 58, 1983.
16. Nomura, T. and Kanzaki, T., Induction of urogenital anomalies and some tumors in the progeny of mice receiving diethylstilbestrol during pregnancy, *Cancer Res.,* 37, 1009, 1977.
17. Nomura, T. and Masuda, M., Carcinogenic and teratogenic activities of diethylstilbestrol in mice, *Life Sci.,* 26, 955, 1980.
18. McLachlan, J. A., Newbold, R. R., and Bullock, B. C., Long-term effects on the female mouse genital tract associated with prenatal exposure to diethylstilbestrol, *Cancer Res.,* 40, 3988, 1980.
19. Walker, B. E., Tumors of female offspring of mice exposed prenatally to diethylstilbestrol, *J. Natl. Cancer Inst.,* 73, 133, 1984.
20. Herbst, A. L., Scully, R. E., Robbey, S. J., Welch, W. R., and Cole, P., Abnormal development of the human genital tract following prenatal exposure to diethylstilbestrol, in *Origins of Human Cancer,* Vol. 4, Hiatt, H. H., Watson, J. D., and Winsten, J. A., Eds., Cold Spring Harbor, New York, 1977, 399.
21. Forsberg, J. C., Developmental mechanism of estrogen-induced irreversible changes in the mouse cervicovaginal epithelium, *J. Natl. Cancer Inst.,* 51, 41, 1979.
22. Weinstein, I. B., The scientific basis for carcinogen detection and primary cancer prevention, *Cancer,* 47, 1133, 1981.
23. McLachlan, J. A., Wong, A., Degen, G. H., and Barrett, J. C., Morphological and neoplastic transformation of Syrian hamster embryo cells by diethylstilbestrol and its analogs, *Cancer Res.,* 42, 3040, 1982.
24. Naylor, P. H., Rabinder, N. K., Loring, J. M., and Villee, C. A., The estrogen-induced/dependent renal adenocarcinoma of the Syrian hamster, in *Regulation of Gene Expression by Hormones,* McKerns, K. W., Ed., Plenum Press, New York, 1983, 39.
25. Li, J. J., Li, S. A., Klicka, J. K., Parsons, J. A., and Lam, L. K. T., Relative carcinogenic activity of various synthetic and natural estrogens in the Syrian hamster kidney, *Cancer Res.,* 43, 5200, 1983.

26. Liehr, J. G., 2-Fluoroestradiol: separation of estrogenicity from carcinogenicity, *Mol. Pharmacol.,* 23, 278, 1983.
27. Li, S. A., Klicka, J. K., and Li, J. J., Estrogen 2- and 4-hydroxylase activity, catechol estrogen formation, and implication for estrogen carcinogenesis in the hamster kidney, *Cancer Res.,* 45, 181, 1985.
28. Liehr, J. G., Modulation of estrogen-induced carcinogenesis by chemical modifications, *Arch. Toxicol.,* 55, 119, 1983.
29. Purdy, R. H., Carcinogenic potential of estrogen in some mammalian model system, *Prog. Cancer Res. Ther.,* 31, 401, 1984.
30. Metzler, M. and McLachlan, J. A., Is diethylstilbestrol bioactivated through peroxidase-mediated oxidation?, *J. Environ. Pathol. Toxicol.,* 1, 531, 1978.
31. Metzler, M. and McLachlan, J. A., The metabolism of diethylstilbestrol, *CRC Crit. Rev. Biochem.,* 10, 171, 1981.
32. Li, J. J. and Li, S. A., High incidence of hepatocellular carcinomas after synthetic estrogen administration in Syrian golden hamsters fed α-naphthoflavone: a new tumor model, *J. Natl. Cancer Inst.,* 73, 543, 1984.
33. Metzler, M., Diethylstilbestrol: reactive metabolites derived from a hormonally active compound, in *Biochemical Basis of Chemical Carcinogenesis,* Greim, H., Jung, K., Karmer, M., Marquardt, H., and Oesch, F., Eds., Raven Press, New York, 1984, 69.
34. Glatt, H. R., Metzler, M., and Oesch, F., Diethylstilbestrol and 11 derivatives: a mutagenicity study with *Salmonella typhimurium, Mutat. Res.,* 67, 113, 1979.
35. Lang, R. and Redmann, U., Non-mutagenicity of some sex hormones in the Ames Salmonella/microsome mutagenicity test, *Mutat. Res.,* 67, 361, 1979.
36. Rudiger, H. W., Haenisch, F., Metzler, M., Oesch, F., and Glatt, H. R., Metabolites of diethylstilbestrol induce sister chromatid exchanges in human cultured fibroblasts, *Nature (London),* 281, 392, 1979.
37. Barrett, J. C., McLachlan, J. A., and Elmore, E., Inability of diethylstilbestrol to induce 6-thioguanine-resistant mutants and to inhibit metabolic cooperation of V79 Chinese hamster cells, *Mutat. Res.,* 107, 427, 1982.
38. Barrett, J. C., Wong, A., and McLachlan, J. A., Diethylstilbestrol induces neoplastic transformation without measurable gene mutation at two loci, *Science,* 212, 1402, 1981.
39. Drevon, C., Piccoli, C., and Montesano, R., Mutagenicity assays of estrogenic hormones in mammalian cells, *Mutat. Res.,* 89, 83, 1981.
40. Kinsella, A. R., Elimination of metabolic co-operation and the induction of sister chromatid exchanges are not properties common to all promoting or co-carcinogenic agents, *Carcinogenesis,* 3, 499, 1982.
41. Myhr, B., Bowers, L., and Caspary, W. J., Assays for the induction of gene mutations at the thymidine kinase locus in L5178Y mouse lymphoma cells in culture, in *Progress in Mutation Research,* Vol. 5, Ashby, J. and deSerres, F. J., Eds., Elsevier, Amsterdam, 1985, 555.
42. Clive, D., Johnson, K. O., Spector, J. F. S., Batson, A. G., and Brown, M. M. M., Validation and characterization of the L5178Y TK$^{+/-}$ mouse lymphoma mutagen assay system, *Mutat. Res.,* 59, 61, 1979.
43. Martin, C. N., McDermid, A. C., and Garner, R. C., Testing of known carcinogens and non-carcinogens for their ability to induce unscheduled DNA synthesis in HeLa cells, *Cancer Res.,* 38, 2621, 1978.
44. Althaus, F. R., Lawrence, S. D., Sattler, G. L., Longfellow, D. G., and Pitot, H. C., Chemical quantification of unscheduled DNA synthesis in cultured hepatocytes as an assay for the rapid screening of potential chemical carcinogens, *Cancer Res.,* 42, 3010, 1982.
45. Hill, A. and Wolff, S., Increased induction of sister chromatid exchange by diethylstilbestrol in lymphocytes from pregnant and premenopausal women, *Cancer Res.,* 42, 893, 1982.
46. Abe, S. and Sasaki, M., Chromosome aberrations and sister chromatid exchanges in Chinese hamster cells exposed to various chemicals, *J. Natl. Cancer Inst.,* 58, 1635, 1977.
47. Tsutsui, T., Degen, G. H., Schiffman, D., Wong, A., Maizumi, H., McLachlan, J. A., and Barrett, J. C., Dependence of exogenous metabolic activation for induction of unscheduled DNA synthesis in Syrian hamster embryo cells by diethylstilbestrol and related compounds, *Cancer Res.,* 44, 184, 1984.
48. Degen, G. H., Wong, A., Eling, T. E., Barrett, J. C., and McLachlan, J. A., Involvement of prostaglandin synthetase in the peroxidative metabolism of diethylstilbestrol in Syrian hamster embryo fibroblast cell cultures, *Cancer Res.,* 43, 992, 1983.
49. Liehr, J. G., Randerath, K., and Randerath, E., Target organ-specific covalent DNA damage preceding diethylstilbestrol-induced carcinogenesis, *Carcinogenesis,* 6, 1067, 1985.
50. Sato, Y., Murai, T., Tsumuraya, M., Saito, H., and Kodama, M., Disruptive effects of diethylstilbestrol on microtubules, *Gann,* 75, 1046, 1984.

51. Sharp, D. C. and Parry, J. M., Diethylstilbestrol: the binding and effects of diethylstilbestrol upon the polymerisation of purified microtubule protein *in vitro, Carcinogenesis,* 6, 865, 1985.
52. Tucker, R. W. and Barrett, J. C., Decreased numbers of spindle and cytoplasmic microtubules in hamster embryo cells treated with a carcinogen, diethylstilbestrol, *Cancer Res.,* 42, 2088, 1986.
53. Kuchler, R. J. and Graver, R. C., Effects of natural estrogens on L strain fibroblasts in tissue culture, *Proc. Soc. Exp. Biol. Med.,* 110, 287, 1982.
54. Rao, P. N. and Engelberg, J., Structural specificity of estrogens in the induction of mitotic chromatid non-disjunction in HeLa cells, *Exp. Cell Res.,* 48, 71, 1967.
55. Lycette, R. R., Whyte, S., and Chapman, C. J., Aneuploid effects of oestradiol on cultured human synovial cells, *N. Z. Med. J.,* 72, 114, 1970.
56. Chrisman, C. L., Aneuploidy in mouse embryos induced by diethylstilbestrol diphosphate, *Teratology,* 9, 229, 1974.
57. Chrisman, C. L. and Hinkle, L. L., Induction of aneuploidy in mouse bone marrow cells with diethylstilbestrol-diphosphate, *Can. J. Genet. Cytol.,* 16, 831, 1974.
58. Chrisman, C. L. and Lasley, J. F., Effects of diethylstilbestrol diphosphate on mitotic activity in bovine lymphocyte cultures, *Cytologia,* 40, 817, 1975.
59. McGaughey, R. W., The culture of pig oocytes in minimal medium, and the influence of progesterone and estradiol-17β on meiotic maturation, *Endocrinology,* 100, 39, 1977.
60. Sawada, M. and Ishidate, M., Jr., Colchicine-like effect of diethylstilbestrol (DES) on mammalian cells *in vitro, Mutat. Res.,* 57, 175, 1978.
61. Parry, J. M., Parry, E. M., and Barrett, J. C., Tumour promoters induce mitotic aneuploidy in yeast, *Nature (London),* 294, 263, 1981.
62. Danford, N. and Parry, J. M., Abnormal cell division in cultured human fibroblasts after exposure to diethylstilbestrol, *Mutat. Res.,* 103, 379, 1982.
63. Tsutsui, T., Maizumi, H., McLachlan, J. A., and Barrett, J. C., Aneuploidy induction and cell transformation by diethylstilbestrol: a possible chromosome mechanism in carcinogenesis, *Cancer Res.,* 43, 3814, 1983.
64. Barrett, J. C., Oshimura, M., Tsutsui, T., and Tanaka, N., Role of aneuploidy in early and late stages of neoplastic progression of Syrian hamster embryo cells in culture, in *Aneuploidy: Etiology and Mechanisms,* Dellarco, V. L., Voytek, P. E., and Hollaender, A., Eds., Plenum Press, New York, 1985, 523.
65. Satya-Prakash, K. L., Hsu, T. C., and Wheeler, W. J., Metaphase arrest, anaphase recovery and aneuploidy induction in cultured Chinese hamster cells following exposure to mitotic arrestants, *Anticancer Res.,* 4, 351, 1984.
66. Pienta, R. J., Transformation of Syrian hamster embryo cells by diverse chemicals and correlation with their reported carcinogenic and mutagenic activities, in *Chemical Mutagens,* Vol. 6, deSerres, F. J., Ed., Plenum Press, New York, 1980, 175.
67. Fu, Y. S., Robboy, S. J., and Prat, J., Nuclear DNA study of vaginal and cervical squamous cell abnormalities in DES-exposed progeny, *J. Obstet. Gynecol.,* 52, 129, 1978.
68. Brand, K. G., Johnson, K. H., and Buoen, L. C., Foreign body tumorigenesis, in *CRC Crit. Rev. Toxicol.,* 4, 353, 1976.
69. Harrington, J. S., Fiber carcinogenesis: epidemiological observations and the Stanton hypothesis, *J. Natl. Cancer Inst.,* 67, 977, 1981.
70. Weisburger, J. H. and Williams, G. M., Carcinogen testing: current problems and new approaches, *Science,* 214, 401, 1981.
71. Mossman, B. T. and Craighead, J. E., Mechanisms of asbestos carcinogenesis, *Environ. Res.,* 25, 269, 1981.
72. Craighead, J. E. and Mossman, B. T., The pathogenesis of asbestos-associated diseases, *N. Engl. J. Med.,* 306, 1446, 1982.
73. Browne, K., Asbestos-related mesothelioma: epidemiological evidence for asbestos as promoter, *Arch. Environ. Health,* 38, 261, 1983.
74. Mossman, B. T., Light, W. G., and Wei, E. T., Asbestos: mechanisms of toxicity and carcinogenicity in the respiratory tract, *Annu. Rev. Pharmacol. Toxicol.,* 23, 595, 1983.
75. Eastman, A., Mossman, B. T., and Bresnick, E., Influence of asbestos on the uptake of benzo(a)pyrene and DNA alkylation in hamster tracheal epithelial cells, *Cancer Res.,* 48, 1251, 1983.
76. Topping, D. C. and Nettesheim, P., Two-stage carcinogenesis studies with asbestos in Fischer 344 rats, *J. Natl. Cancer Inst.,* 65, 627, 1980.
77. Topping, D. C., Nettesheim, P., and Martin, D. H., Toxic and tumorigenic effects of asbestos on tracheal mucosa, *J. Environ. Pathol. Toxicol.,* 3, 261, 1980.
78. Stanton, M. F., Layard, M., Tegeris, A., Miller, E., May, M., and Kent, E., Carcinogenicity of fibrous glass: pleural response in the rat in relation to fiber dimension, *J. Natl. Cancer Inst.,* 58, 587, 1977.

79. Wagner, J. C., Berry, G., and Timbrell, V., Mesotheliomata in rats after innoculation with asbestos and other materials, *Br. J. Cancer,* 28, 173, 1973.

80. Wagner, J. C., Berry, G., Skidmore, J. W., and Timbrell, V., The effects of the inhalation of asbestos in rats, *Br. J. Cancer,* 29, 252, 1974.

81. Hesterberg, T. W. and Barrett, J. C., Dependence of asbestos- and mineral dust-induced transformation of mammalian cells in culture on fiber dimension, *Cancer Res.,* 44, 2170, 1984.

82. Lechner, J. F., Tokiwa, T., LaVeck, M., Benedict, W. F., Banks-Schlegel, S., Yeager, H., Baneijee, A., and Harris, C. C., Asbestos-associated chromosomal changes in human mesothelial cells, *Proc. Natl. Acad. Sci. U.S.A.,* 82, 3884, 1985.

83. Paterour, J. J., Bignon, J., and Jaurand, M. J., *In vitro* transformation of rat pleural mesothelial cells by chrysotile fibers and/or benzo(a)pyrene, *Carcinogenesis,* 6, 523, 1985.

84. Poole, A., Brown, R. C., Turner, C. J., Skidmore, J. W., and Griffiths, D. M., *In vitro* genotoxic activities of fibrous erionite, *Br. J. Cancer,* 47, 697, 1983.

85. Oshimura, M., Hesterberg, T. W., Tsutsui, T., and Barrett, J. C., Correlation of asbestos-induced cytogenetic effects with cell transformation of Syrian hamster embryo cells in culture, *Cancer Res.,* 44, 5017, 1984.

86. Sincock, A. M. and Seabright, M., Induction of chromosome changes in Chinese hamster cells by exposure to asbestos fibers, *Nature (London),* 257, 56, 1975.

87. Hesterberg, T. W. and Barrett, J. C., Induction by asbestos fibers of anaphase abnormalities: mechanism for aneuploidy induction and possibly carcinogenesis, *Carcinogenesis,* 6, 473, 1985.

88. Rachko, D. and Brand, K. G., Chromosomal aberrations in foreign body tumorigenesis in mice, *Proc. Soc. Exp. Biol. Med.,* 172, 382, 1983.

89. Boone, C. W., Takeichi, N., Ande Eaton, S., and Paranjpe, M., "Spontaneous" neoplastic transformation *in vitro:* a form of foreign body (smooth surface) tumorigenesis, *Science,* 204, 177, 1979.

90. Williams, G. M., DNA reactive and epigenetic carcinogens, in *Mechanisms of Environmental Carcinogenesis,* Vol. 1, Barrett, J. C., Ed., CRC Press, Boca Raton, Fla., 1987, chap. 7.

91. International Agency for Research on Cancer, Monograph on the Evaluation of the Carcinogenic Risk of Chemicals to Humans, Suppl. 4, IARC, London, 1982, 50.

92. Ashby, J., deSerres, F. J., Draper, M., Ishidate, M., Margolin, B. H., Matter, B. E., and Shelby, M. D., *Evaluation of Short-Term Tests for Carcinogens,* Elsevier, Amsterdam, 1985.

93. Lee, T. C., Oshimura, M., and Barrett, J. C., Comparison of arsenic-induced cell transformation cytotoxicity, mutation and chromosome effects in Syrian hamster embryo cells in culture, *Carcinogenesis,* 6, 1421, 1985.

94. Waters, M. D., Genetic toxicology of some known or suspected human carcinogens, in *Chemical Mutagens,* deSerres, F. J., Ed., Plenum Press, New York, 1984, 261.

95. Squibb, K. S. and Fowler, B. A., The toxicity of arsenic and its compounds, in *Biological and Environmental Effects of Arsenic,* Fowler, B. A., Ed., Elsevier, Amsterdam, 1983, 133.

96. Tkeshelashvilli, L. K., Shearman, C. W., Zakour, R. A., Koplitz, R. M., and Loeb, L. A., Effects of arsenic, selenium and chromium on the fidelity of DNA synthesis, *Cancer Res.,* 40, 2455, 1980.

97. Tsutsui, T., Maizumi, H., and Barrett, J. C., Colcemid-induced neoplastic transformation and aneuploidy in Syrian hamster embryo cells, *Carcinogenesis,* 5, 89, 1984.

98. International Agency for Research on Cancer, Some anti-thyroid and related substances, nitro-furans and industrial chemicals, Monographs on the Evaluation of Carcinogenic Risk of Chemicals to Man, Vol. 7, IARC, Lyon, 1974, 31.

99. Tsutsui, T., Maizumi, H., and Barrett, J. C., Amitrole-induced cell transformation and gene mutations in Syrian hamster embryo cells in culture, *Mutat. Res.,* 140, 205, 1984.

100. Report of ICPEMC Task Group 5 on the differentiation between genotoxic and non-genotoxic carcinogens, *Mutat. Res.,* 133, 1, 1984.

101. Jones, P. A., Role of DNA methylation in regulating gene expression, differentiation, and carcinogenesis, in *Mechanisms of Environmental Carcinogenesis,* Vol. 1, Barrett, J. C., Ed., CRC Press, Boca Raton, Fla., 1987, chap. 2.

102. Bruce, S. A., Gyi, K. K., Nakano, S., Ueo, H., Zajac-Kaye, M., and Ts'o, P. O. P., Genetic and developmental determinants in neoplastic transformation, in *Biochemical Basis of Chemical Carcinogenesis,* Griem, H., Jung, R., Kramer, K., Harquardt, H., and Oesch, F., Eds., Raven Press, New York, 1984, 159.

103. Benedict, W. F., Banerjee, A., Gardner, A., and Jones, P. A., Induction of morphological transformation in mouse C3H 10T$_{1/2}$ clone 8 cells and chromosomal damage in hamster A(T$_1$)C1-3 cells by cancer chemotherapeutic agents, *Cancer Res.,* 37, 2202, 1977.

104. Reddy, J. K., Azarnoff, D. L., and Hignite, C. E., Hypolipidemic hepatic peroxisome proliferators form a novel class of chemical carcinogens, *Nature (London),* 283, 397, 1980.

105. Fahl, W. E., Lalwani, N. D., Watanabe, T., Goel, S. K., and Reddy, J. K., DNA damage related to increased hydrogen peroxide generation by hypolipidemic drug-induced liver peroxisomes, *Proc. Natl. Acad. Sci. U.S.A.,* 81, 7827, 1984.

106. Popp, J. A., Garvey, L. K., Hamm, T. E., Jr., and Swenberg, J. A., Lack of hepatic promotional activity by the peroxisomal proliferating hepatic carcinogen di(2-ethylhexyl)phthalate, *Carcinogenesis*, 6, 141, 1985.

107. Butterworth, B. E., Bermudez, E., Smith-Oliver, T., Earle, L., Cattley, R., Martin, J., Popp, J. A., Stram, S., Jirtle, R., and Michalopoulos, G., Lack of genotoxic activity of di(2-ethylhexyl)phthalate (DEHP) in rat and human hepatocytes, *Carcinogenesis*, 5, 1329, 1984.

108. Phillips, B. J., James, T. E. B., and Gangolli, S. D., Genotoxocity studies of di(2-ethylhexyl)phthalate and its metabolites in CHO cells, *Mutat. Res.*, 102, 297, 1982.

109. Carter, T. H., The regulation of gene expression by tumor promoters, in *Mechanisms of Environmental Carcinogenesis*, Vol. 1, Barrett, J. C., Ed., CRC Press, Boca Raton, Fla., 1987, chap. 4.

110. Colburn, N. H., The genetics of tumor promotion, in *Mechanisms of Environmental Carcinogenesis*, Vol. 1, Barrett, J. C., Ed., CRC Press, Boca Raton, Fla., 1987, chap. 5.

111. Boutwell, R. K., The function and mechanism of promoters of carcinogenesis, *CRC Crit. Rev. Toxicol.*, 2, 419, 1974.

112. Scott, W. T. and Watanabe, P. G., Differentiation of genetic versus epigenetic mechanisms of toxicity and its application to risk assessment, *Drug Metab. Rev.*, 13, 853, 1982.

113. Pitot, H. C., Goldsworthy, T., and Moran, S., The natural history of carcinogenesis: implications of experimental carcinogenesis in the genesis of human cancer, *J. Supramol. Struct. Cell. Biochem.*, 17, 133, 1981.

114. Hecker, E., Structure-activity relationships in diterpene esters irritant and cocarcinogenic to mouse skin, in *Carcinogenesis*, Vol. 2, Slaga, T. J., Sivak, A., and Boutwell, R. K., Eds., Raven Press, New York, 1978, 11.

115. Scribner, J. and Suss, R., Tumor initiation and promotion, in *International Review of Experimental Pathology*, Richter, G. W. and Epstein, M. A., Eds., Academic Press, New York, 1978, 137.

116. Copeland, E. S., Free radicals in promotion — a chemical pathology study section workshop, *Cancer Res.*, 43, 5631, 1983.

117. Cerutti, P., Prooxidant states and tumor promotion, *Science*, 227, 375, 1985.

118. Rao, P. M., Rajalakshmi, A. A., Sarma, D. S. R., Pala, M., and Parodi, S., Orotic acid, a promoter of liver carcinogenesis induces DNA damage in rat liver, *Carcinogenesis*, 6, 765, 1985.

119. Hennings, H., Tumor promotion and progression in mouse skin, in *Mechanisms of Environmental Carcinogenesis*, Vol. 2, Barrett, J. C., Ed., CRC Press, Boca Raton, Fla., 1987, chap. 11.

120. Ronen, A., 2-Aminopurine, *Mutat. Res.*, 75, 1, 1979.

121. Sugiura, K., Teller, M. N., Parham, J. C., and Brown, G. B., A comparison of the oncogenicities of 3-hydroxyxanthine, guanine 3-N-oxide, and some related compounds, *Cancer Res.*, 30, 184, 1970.

122. Trainin, N., Kaye, A. M., and Berenblum, I., Influence of mutagens on the initiation of skin carcinogenesis, *Biochem. Pharmacol.*, 13, 263, 1964.

123. Barrett, J. C., Somatic mutation and neoplastic transformation of mammalian cells induced by two modified purines, 2-aminopurine and 6-N-hydroxylaminopurine, *Proc. Natl. Acad. Sci. U.S.A.*, 75, 3297, 1981.

124. Freese, E. B., The mutagenic effect of hydroxyaminopurine derivatives on phage T_4, *Mutat. Res.*, 5, 299, 1968.

125. Brockman, H. E. and deSerres, F. J., Induction of *ad-3* mutants of *Neurospora crassa* by 2-aminopurine, *Genetics*, 48, 596, 1963.

126. Brockman, H. E., deSerres, F. J., and Ong, T. M., Potent mutagenicity of 6-N-hydroxyl-amino purine and 2-amino-N^6-hydroxyadenine at the *ad-3* region of *Neurospora crassa*, in Proc. of Environmental Mutagenic Society 10th Annual Meeting, 1979, 55a.

127. Tsutsui, T., Maizumi, H., and Barrett, J. C., Induction by modified purines (2-aminopurine and 6-N-hydroxylaminopurine) of chromosome aberrations and aneuploidy in Syrian hamster embryo cells, *Mutat. Res.*, 148, 107, 1984.

128. Shelby, M. D. and Stasiewicz, S., Chemicals showing no evidence of carcinogenicity in long-term, two species rodent studies: the need for short-term test data, *Environ. Mutagen.*, 6, 871, 1984.

129. Zeiger, E. and Tennant, R. W., Mutagenesis, clastogenesis, carcinogenesis: expectations, correlations and relations, in *Genetic Toxicology of Environmental Chemicals, Part B: Genetic Effects and Applied Mutagenesis*, Ramel, C., Lambert, B., and Magnussen, J., Eds., Alan R. Liss, New York, 1986, 75.

130. Toman, Z., Dambly, C., and Radman, M., Induction of a stable, heritable epigenetic change by mutagenic carcinogens: a new test system, *IARC Sci. Publ.*, 27, 243, 1980.

131. Oshimura, M., unpublished data.

132. International Agency for Research on Cancer, Approaches to Classifying Chemical Carcinogens According to Mechanism of Action, Intern. Tech. Rep. No. 83001, IARC, Lyon, 1983.

INDEX

M

N

O